Charles Stewart Loch

How to Help Cases of Distress

A Handy Reference Book for Almoners and Others

Charles Stewart Loch

How to Help Cases of Distress
A Handy Reference Book for Almoners and Others

ISBN/EAN: 9783337416447

Printed in Europe, USA, Canada, Australia, Japan

Cover: Foto ©Lupo / pixelio.de

More available books at **www.hansebooks.com**

HOW TO HELP CASES OF DISTRESS

A HANDY REFERENCE BOOK FOR

ALMONERS AND OTHERS

BY

C. S. LOCH

SECRETARY TO THE COUNCIL
OF
THE CHARITY ORGANISATION SOCIETY, LONDON

FIFTH EDITION
JUNE 1895

LONDON
CHARITY ORGANISATION SOCIETY, 15 BUCKINGHAM STREET, STRAND, W.C.
AND
LONGMANS, GREEN, & CO., PATERNOSTER ROW

PRINTED BY
SPOTTISWOODE AND CO., NEW-STREET SQUARE
LONDON

PREFACE.

THIS book is a reprint of the Introduction to the 'Charities Register and Digest,' the fourth edition of which has been published this year. In the Register will be found very complete information in regard to Charitable Institutions available for the metropolis. In an Appendix attached to it are given particulars in regard to Provident, Friendly, and Trade Societies, and Savings Banks.[1]

In this, the Introduction, the attempt is made to furnish such general information as a person desirous of assisting those in distress would wish to have at hand. Many are ignorant of the powers and functions of our public authorities in the administration of relief, and overlook the large and complicated machinery which the community has from time to time created for that purpose. To them an account of the duties and responsibilities of these authorities, and of the machinery which has been placed at their disposal, may be of service. On the other hand, to many who are more or less skilled in the administration of relief a short book of reference, which is written from their own point of view, and deals only with the facts with which they are primarily concerned, may be useful for consultation.

The selection of subjects in this book is based on the needs of every-day practical charitable work. A case of distress might be cited as a reason for almost every paragraph.

[1] For the Table of Contents of the Register see p. ccvi at the end of this volume.

Readers desirous of further information are urged to refer to the books mentioned in the list on page cxcvi. These, with other publications on charitable questions, can be seen at the offices of the Council of the Society.

The Table of Contents has been enlarged and the Index omitted. It has been thought that, as the book is written in short sections, any particular point may, after consulting the Contents, be found with sufficient precision by reference to the section in which it is likely to be mentioned.

For this edition a very large part of ' the Introduction ' has been re-written, and care has been taken to introduce notes on the many new Acts of Parliament that have been passed during the last five years and bear more or less closely on the work of an almoner.

C. S. L.

June 1895.

CONTENTS.

INTRODUCTION.

INTRODUCTION.[1]

I.—THE SCOPE OF THE INTRODUCTION.

THIS 'Introduction' is rather a reference book than an introductory preface. A list of charities, without some knowledge of the modes in which their benefits ought to be turned to account, is like a pharmacopœia without a knowledge of the elements of medicine. An outline of the principles of charitable work has therefore been given. Legislation also has created public bodies with definite responsibilities, which, if properly fulfilled, narrow the field of charity. At present there is a mingling of obligations and an overlapping of responsibility. A division of labour would add to the efficacy of charity; but before this becomes possible, those who take an interest in these questions (and in some way or other most people are dealing with them) must learn what public authorities have to do, and how their resources can be made use of with the greatest advantage to the poorer classes. For this reason particulars have been inserted in the Introduction in regard to the Poor Law, Reformatory and Industrial Schools, the vestries and their sanitary duties, &c. &c.[2] As the object of charity is to

[1] The Introduction may be had separately, price 2s. 6d.

[2] With regard to the necessary limits under which this information is given, see note p. xlv. A list of books for reference and reading, and a list of some of the publications of the Charity Organisation Society, will be found on p. cxcv.

N.B.—It is particularly requested that any corrections, information regarding new or omitted charities, and suggestions with regard to the improvement of the Charities Register and Digest, and of this Introduction in future editions, be sent to the Secretary, Charity Organisation Society, 15 Buckingham Street, London, W.C.

Persons desirous of assisting cases of distress of a difficult nature are invited to refer to the same address, should they be unable to find for them a suitable mode of help in the Register, or if they cannot ascertain from the Introduction the information they require.

Necessity of a knowledge of methods of charitable work and of legal provisions.

a

benefit the individual and his family, and the attainment of this object depends on the discrimination of circumstances and the application of remedies, typical instances of various classes of cases have been given; *e.g.* widows with families, the unemployed, chronic cases, inebriates. These are, generally speaking, intended as illustrations of what cases may rightly be left to public bodies and what should be undertaken by charity.

The 'Introduction' does not deal with those social and economic questions, which lie partly within and partly without the province of charity—in what ways the conditions which tend to the degradation of life in large sections of the people may be removed. Such questions must repeatedly occur to every one who has any experience in, or has given any thought to, the relief of individuals. But though they be most important, and though the study of them in connection with a knowledge of the daily life of the people be a chief duty of our time, yet, except incidentally, they lie beyond the scope of this work.

II.—Explanatory of the Register.

The scope of the Register is larger than that usually aimed at in such works. This is mainly due to the introduction of information in regard to the various provident agencies, a knowledge of which is of the first importance to the almoner. And also the attempt has been made to give prominence to those large charities of the working classes which are habitually overlooked, but which are administered with a familiar acquaintance with the general circumstances of the recipients, and have a potency for good which may greatly exceed the more distant though equally genuine charities of other classes. Charity is of no class and of no sect; it has to prevent, to remedy, and not merely to alleviate distress; every spiritual and material agency that has this purpose or can be so utilised is its minister: for those who are in distress it has to open the way to sober living, health, and self-support, and, so far as it is both wise and strong, for their children's children. It is with this idea that the Register has been compiled.

To refer to the Register it will be well in every case to consult the index first. The entries in the index refer to classes of charities, to individual charities, to the places at which institutions are, and to those names which are commonly used as short titles of well-known institutions, *e.g.* the Boxhill Convalescent Home, the Strangers' Friend Society (otherwise called the Benevolent Society), &c. Of the religious charities only an alphabetical list has been given. Those which combine religious and material work are entered twice, and full particulars are given in regard to the latter. Those that are engaged in religious work only (with some very important exceptions, such as the City Mission, the Parochial Mission-women Fund, of which more lengthy entries have been inserted), are concerned with evangelisation abroad, or have special objects which do not come within the ordinary cognizance of the almoner. The entries of the material charities show (1) the name and object, (2) the mode of admission, (3) the management, (4) the number of persons benefited, and (5) the income. The second head is the most important to the almoner. Under it he will find details of the exact conditions under which each institution will deal with cases, and the class of case which it takes. The almoner will thus be able to classify cases for himself, ascertaining without correspondence with institutions, and hence without expense and delay, whether they are or are not suitable.

The lists of charities for the Blind, Deaf and Dumb, Reformatory and Industrial Schools, Training Ships, Boarding-out Committees and Schools for Children, Training and other Homes for Girls, Institutions for Idiots and Imbeciles, Convalescent Homes, have been made as complete as possible—including institutions which are not metropolitan.

The thanks of the Council of the Charity Organisation Society are due to the very large number of persons who have co-operated in the production of this work, and to whom the Council is indebted both for information and suggestions.

It has been found convenient to use the word almoner throughout this Introduction. Many persons give up time to almsgiving. They are those whom questions of the administration of charity most closely affect, and on whose capacity and intelligence its beneficence largely depends ; yet, as almost all have some part in this work, the word should be taken in its widest sense.

III.—CHARITIES LISTS GENERALLY.

Before passing to the functions of charity, the Poor Law, and other subjects, a word of recognition is due to those who have been forerunners in this work. The late Mr. Samuel Gurney, it would appear from his paper at the London meeting of the Congrès de Bienfaisance in 1862, had commenced a Register of Charities. He says [1] that he had begun a register the object of which was 'to enable the benevolent,' by means of authentic data, 'to investigate for themselves, either briefly or fully, the workings of the various charities of the metropolis, or to ascertain without trouble the institutions suited to the special circumstances of cases in which

[1] Quoted in the Annual Report of the Council of the Charity Organisation Society, 1879, p. 15.

they are interested.' The late Dr. Hawksley's well-known paper on the London Charities (1868) pointed significantly to the necessity of more general knowledge on the whole subject. Mr. G. M. Hicks compiled a most elaborate tabular statement of some of the London charities, which was published in the 'Times' in 1869; his continued interest in the subject, and his subsequent notes upon it, which showed that weighty conclusions might be drawn from a careful analysis of the reports of institutions, have encouraged in their task those who have been entrusted with the compilation of this Register. And the successively published Annual Guide-books of Messrs. Fry, Low, and Howe have all been of service in turning attention to the large number and various kinds of charitable institutions in the metropolis; and some editions of the second especially contained, with a plan of classification, much detailed information which was most valuable. 'The Charities Register and Digest' of the Charity Organisation Society has grown out of the wants of the Society. Frequent inquiries were and are made of it in regard to the action and merits of institutions; a manuscript register was commenced for purposes of reference in 1879. It was found that its usefulness would be greatly increased if it were printed. At the same time the want of some book of reference in regard to conditions of admission to the benefits of institutions and societies was widely felt in the District Committees of the Society. The plan of the Register was therefore altered to its present form, and its compilation was commenced in 1881.[1]

IV.—THE PRINCIPLES OF CHARITY.

Truism as it may appear, it is very necessary to say in the first place, that charity unwisely administered is capable of doing incalculable harm to its recipients. Almsgiving or charity is, properly speaking, the rendering of service to another out of love or pity. The pressure of the 'wholesome urgencies of life' is a condition of moral and physical sanity. The individual should provide against hunger,

---

[1] It may be mentioned that in the preparation of the last edition of the Register the Society had the assistance of Mr. R. B. Prosser, to whom the credit of many improvements in its compilation is due. Mr. R. Hepburn has edited this, the 1895, edition, with the assistance of several sub-editors. Mr. H. J. Wilson, the Secretary to the Gardner's Trust for the Blind, has had charge of the section relating to that class. Miss Poole, the Secretary to the Metropolitan Association for Befriending Young Servants, has supervised the revision of the sections relating to Homes, especially those for girls and young women. Mr. C. H. Baker, the Assistant Secretary to the Church Penitentiary Association, has revised and enlarged the section 'Penitents.' In the section relating to Hospitals and Dispensaries, which has been recast and, it is believed, greatly improved, the Society has had the advantage of very useful expert assistance. Much care has been taken to include in the Register the latest available information respecting Endowed Charities.

nakedness, and want of shelter; the father against these things both for himself and his wife and family. The ordinary contingencies of life, which fall within the range of ordinary foresight, should, for the individual's own sake and for society's sake, be met by the efforts of the individual. Charity which, for love or pity's sake, seduces the individual from the wise and natural toilsomeness of life, or which does not induce him to bear the burden, by helping him to overcome his weakness and pushing him forward to self-maintenance, is, under the cloak, real or assumed, of love and pity, the poor man's greatest foe—greatest because it comes like an angel of loving-kindness, and yet produces far-reaching woe like a spirit of evil.

Next we would draw attention to a distinction which Burke drew between the poor and the indigent. The former are those wage-earners who are the real wealth-creators of the community. They are well, and should, so far as material charity is concerned, be left alone. Bad charity tends to tempt them into the indigent class; good charity, if they are in distress, prevents their falling into that class. The indigent are those who are habitually in want; good charity with adequate help raises them to self-support; bad charity with intermittent, purposeless help degrades them to ever lower degradation.

Consider the matter economically, commercially, socially, and religiously. Every one in the indigent class represents a deficit. His keep, if the whole period of his life and his recognised individual responsibilities are taken into account, is more than his earnings: the difference in some way or other is made up by his neighbours—by charity or a poor's-rate; or if it is not made up, there is, to use a medical term, a decline or consumption. Not maintained in these ways, he is underfed, underclad, insanitarily housed, and sinks to weakness and inability to work. If he has children, the evils pass to them and subsequent generations. Obviously, therefore, economically the indigent are a ' dead loss ' to the community.

Next consider the matter commercially. There is indigence—much indigence—due to physical and mental weakness, to weakness of character and feebleness of purpose. But some methods of employment aggravate these tendencies; some diminish them. Intermittent employment, which no doubt cannot be wholly dispensed with, has the former result. It may be caused by the exigencies of the labour market, or by the necessary slackness of many kinds of employment in the winter months. Each of these causes suggests a different remedy—and in each, so far as a remedy is forthcoming, indigence will be lessened.

Take the former cause first—intermittent employment due to the varying exigencies of the labour market. This tends to make men work hard, sometimes excessively hard, for days or weeks, leaving them idle and listless afterwards; till pressure rouses them to seek work elsewhere, or a new job turns up. It makes them careless or, at least, unmindful of the future; and sometimes they seem to have no sense of its obligations at all. Some are disheartened by failure; others relapse into an easy-going dependence, of which one sign is 'a horror of hard work' and an extraordinary shiftiness in finding excuses so as to avoid it. It is natural that those who belong to the lowest ranks in our labour market should gravitate to centres where they have a chance of obtaining work on demand. To take the Docks as an illustration. Much of the labour at the Docks is adept labour—it requires strength and knack, or skill. Those who have these qualifications are more likely to obtain employment than others. They are therefore less likely to be indigent. But as adaptability and strength decrease, indigence is more likely to supervene, even if personal faults and weaknesses do not drag the individual down. This indigence, due often to the lessened adaptability and strength which is felt at a comparatively early period of life—a life in which the pressure is sometimes tense, sometimes almost nil—can only be guarded against by regularity of employment, as dock and other authorities have recently been learning, even if the boon be purchased by a lower wage. This lower wage may be but the higher wages earned intermittently throughout the year reduced to an average, and may seem, by comparison, small when contrasted with the wages earned in particular weeks, as, for instance, when an unusually large number of hands are required at a wool sale. But its regularity is a sufficient compensation for this comparative smallness; and to systematise work and thus employ, with as much regularity as possible, an average number at an average wage is to prevent indigence.

Next, with regard to the intermittent work of the winter. The effect of a cause such as this, which is due to the very seasons themselves, can hardly be modified, except so far as men undertake different kinds of work at different times in the year; and probably comparatively few do this. There is therefore, in most instances, only one way out of the difficulty. Where, again, personal faults and weaknesses do not drag the individual down, he may be protected by a trade combination, or he may protect himself. If he is in an union, he may have out-of-work pay at about 10s. a week. If he is not in an union, he may average his own pay, so that from the summer he may carry enough over to last him through the two months or so of lessened work in the winter. But as a rule the persons who suffer from the winter's pressure are labourers or unskilled workmen who belong to trades for which there are no strong unions; or they are, for instance, men who are painters, but not painters indeed, who have never served an apprenticeship, and who are disqualified from joining any trade society. Hence, in their case, if indigence is to be avoided, they must become a rule to themselves and average their own wage. But again, in regard to winter slackness, too, it may be said that, so far as work can be systematised so as to equalise the differences of demand due to the difference of the season, indigence will be prevented. On what principle each man will apply his wage each must be the judge. But any system by which intermittent labour is needlessly employed is injurious to the community.

Those who are employed intermittently, if they do not by trade organisation or personal contrivance fill in the blanks of the year, when employment is slack, by drawing on their stock of savings, must become the 'corner men' of life. They do not live on air: they live at the cost of others, on their wives and on their children. They borrow and live on credit. Sometimes they exact toll of their comrades in pence and pots of beer; sometimes they beg; sometimes they are on short commons, underfed or well-nigh starved. So far as their services are of any value, the community loses their unexpended labour and their unearned wage. Thus, commercially, it is to the interest of the community, and indirectly of each business man, that there should be as few indigent persons as possible. Charity or relief is often, in fact, an insufficient and wasteful self-imposed tax on the part of the more regularly employed population to compensate for these 'deficits,' which the unfitness of the labourer for work requiring strength, knack, or skill, his personal faults and weaknesses, combined with the rigour of competition and an imperfect industrial organisation, tend to create. Thus, out of intermittent labour spring many woes. It produces intermittent energy; the off-days become habitual; with indolence comes intemperance; with uncertainty of employment comes recklessness about the future; from these result pauperism, and the whole series of mental and physical infirmities which are features of pauperism. If these are the results, viewed economically and commercially, those who know how the good of 'the masses' is but, stated in another way, the good of the individual—powerful to influence neighbours by example in all smaller domestic and personal matters, and intelligent in the choice of councillors, 'guardians,' and other representatives—will see that indigence is also a social evil.

With regard to it religiously—to pass by many urgent witnesses, it has been said: 'On all sides, in the most degraded localities, physically and morally, we find ourselves surrounded with religious agencies busying themselves in attending to the higher interests of the masses in the most devoted manner, and at great outlay. Bitter complaints have been made as to the poverty of the results obtained by such multifarious and strenuous endeavours. This need be no wonder, when we reflect on the overwhelming dis-

advantage against which the missionary and philanthropist have to
contend. Our poor are so lodged, that to inhale the atmosphere in their
houses is enough to produce a lethargic depression, to escape from
which is but to be exposed to the temptations of the High Street and
Cowgate. With no comfort at home, the poor labourer is forced to
go elsewhere for enjoyment. To his sleeping-place he returns to
find himself in a crowded apartment, where is no attempt to maintain the ordinary decencies of life. With so many and varied
proclivities to vice in all its forms it is a heartless task to talk to
such a one of "righteousness, temperance, and judgment to come."[1]

On all grounds, therefore, to prevent distress from lapsing into
habitual indigence, to create safeguards against indigence, and to
rescue from indigence, is the *interest*—to put it at the lowest inducement—of every one in the community, whatever his vocation,
business, or personal views about politics or religion. What has
been said will, we trust, give a glimpse of the tracts of work which
lie alongside of the work of charity, and to which the thoughts of
all who would not ' *kill* with kindness' must frequently pass.

What, then, are the principles of charity—that charity which
will lessen misery, not merely without weakening, but by producing,
self-reliance, which will do kind acts and yet not diminish the energy
or impair the character and morality of the people? The subsequent sections of this introduction are an answer to this question.
But it may be well to state these principles here, omitting for
brevity's sake some modifying conditions and reservations. (1)
As a rule, no work of charity is complete which does not place the
person benefited in self-dependence. Obviously if this principle is
true, the administration of most of our charitable institutions must be
altered; many must be reorganised. All gifts and all forms of
relief should be but parts of a treatment having self-dependence
and recovery from distress as its end. Relief given practically to
all comers, without reference to the whole of the circumstances of
the individual, is given at haphazard, and is injurious. Charity
should abandon such relief and become a partner, as it were, in the
work of thrift. There is now no such partnership. Conveniences
and opportunities and possibilities for thrift and saving exist, but
charity does not use them. There is no organised relation between
the two. (2) All means of pressure, such as the fear of destitution, a sense of shame, the influence of relatives, must be brought
to bear, or left to act upon the individual. He must, as far as
possible, be thrown on his own resources. (3) In deciding whether
relief should or should not be given, or what assistance should
be provided, the family must be taken as a whole; otherwise
the strongest social bond will be weakened. Family obligations—

---

[1] ' Report on the Sanitary Condition of Edinburgh,' by Dr. H. J. Littlejohn. 1866.

care for the aged, responsibility for the young, help in sickness and trouble—should be cast, so far as possible, on the family. (4) Further, as material charity is only a part, and a small part, of efficacious charity, a thorough knowledge is necessary both of the circumstances of the persons to be benefited and the means of aiding them ; and the element of personal influence and control must very largely predominate over the monetary and eleemosynary element. At present this is out of all proportion small. (5) The relief, to effect a cure, must be suitable in kind and adequate in quantity. The individual treatment of individual cases on a definite plan, and with sufficient knowledge, is a *sine quâ non* in beneficial almsgiving. Charity also must learn to require just terms of its beneficiaries. It must consider them not as recipients of gifts, but men and women whose standard of life has to be raised. The truest charity often lies in the righteous fulfilment of duty, whether personal or public ; and next to it must often be placed that charity which is vigilant to see duty done. Charity that fulfils the natural duties of others is in the main a wrong and deceptive charity. Charity that helps others to do their duty is the most genuine and salutary, as it is the most difficult, charity.

V.— On the Responsibility of the Charitable, and Methods of Charity.

We have for convenience' sake considered those in distress either as the indigent who are habitually in want, or as those who can be saved or rescued from indigence. The former, making allowance, of course, for special circumstances in each individual instance, we may call, for want of a better word, ineligible for charity— the latter eligible. In England there is State charity, or at least a State fund for the destitute: it rightly deals with the indigent. Subject, therefore, to considerations to be afterwards dealt with, charity can, without fear of consequences, limit its scope to the curable. It may be said that the Poor Law does its work with a want of uniformity, and at best but indifferently well: if so it should be improved, and not superseded, by charity. But the true position of charitable work remains intact. All eligible cases should properly be dealt with by it. But how can a distinction be drawn ? By no other plan than either a thorough personal acquaintance with the history and circumstances of those in distress, which is possible only when there has been long-continued familiar intercourse or frequent and sufficient contact with them and people of the same type ; or by an inquiry which, combined with personal experience, may be a satisfactory substitute for this. It will hardly be said that the former method is possible, unless in a very few exceptional instances, in London or large towns : it is very

Cases eligible for charity : cases ineligible.

often impossible even in the country. We must content ourselves therefore with considering what is the best substitute. Rich and poor do not live in the same quarter of the town; even if they did, social distinctions and interests would much divide them; each cannot pretend to know much about the other: individuals no doubt may make inroads into 'poor districts,' or the poorer quarters of well-to-do neighbourhoods, but they seldom make a chief purpose of their life the acquisition of a knowledge of the facts of social life by their own personal observation in conjunction with charitable work. Separated by birth and education, if not by residence, they seldom become members, as it were, of the same community. Class differences remain, though class distinctions may be softened, obliterated, and altogether forgotten in good-will. Yet, however serious these difficulties may be, the obligation of the almoner remains the same. Whoever gives charitable aid undertakes a definite responsibility : he is not, for instance, entitled to injure the person he thinks he will help. To make sure that he does not, he must learn all the circumstances, on a consideration of which he will decide whether or how he can help effectually. We may even put it more strongly—he has no right to interfere, unless he justifies his interference not merely by a well-meaning but by a *Inquiry.* well-directed charity. Inquiry then is the acquisition of such information as may make charity productive of good results. Two kinds of knowledge are required for the purpose : a knowledge of particular facts and of the social life of the class of which the person in distress is a member (for this purpose the services of an inquiry officer may be desirable), and a general knowledge of character—combined with a discernment of the value of evidence, and a knowledge of the modes and possibilities of charitable assistance (for this purpose a well-educated and instructed almoner is a *sine quâ non*). And to check the individual judgment, which it is always necessary to do, there should be a committee, especially a committee containing members of all classes and having all kinds of influence and special knowledge. Many have no aptitude for almoner's work ; none can do it to good purpose without study and training. Doctors have to be educated methodically, registered, and certificated. Charity is the work of the social physician. It is to the interest of the community that it should not be entrusted to novices or to *dilettanti*, or to quacks.

The scope of the inquiry which usually is necessary may be indicated by the following heads, on which usually information must be obtained :—(1) The parents ; earnings at the time of application and previously ; cause of leaving last employ ; their children ; the ages of parents and children ; whether the children go to school, and, if so, where ; or, if they are employed, what they earn. (2) The previous addresses of the family. (3) Their references. (4) Whether they belong to a club, or have relations who ought to assist. (5) What debts they have; and what their rent is. (6) How they are obtaining a living at the time of application, and how they think they can be thoroughly helped.

Then follows the investigation on this basis : to learn the cause of distress ; to verify ; to search out the best mode of helping; to throw a fair share of the burden of assistance on relatives ; by visiting the home, and in other ways to ascertain the character of the family ; to learn on whom, if the head of the family lacks force of character or is weak, reliance can be placed to re-establish the family fortunes ; to settle what means of future thrift and self-support can be organised. A sympathetic and thorough investigation will elicit facts on all these points. Upon them the committee will then have to decide. We say 'the committee,' but if a private almoner can spare the time to work in this fashion and has the necessary resources at his command, the ends of charity will be equally gained. Yet single-handed he cannot effect so much as he will if associated with others.

Investigation, then, will indicate who are the curable, and will limit the field of charity, as apart from that of the Poor Law and other public bodies.

To these statements one or two objections may be made. Objections to inquiry considered. Inquiry will check enthusiasm and devotion, it may be said. Facts prove the contrary. Inquiry startles the novice as a revelation of new knowledge ; but it gives him eventually a security in his work, which imposes on him many restrictions, and requires of him perpetual thoughtfulness, but which is as a high road compared with the fool's paradise in which he formerly walked boldly along. Inquiry, also, throws into prominence the imperative necessity of nourishing and bringing into operation all the finer elements of charity—personal influence, a long-suffering patience, a quick sympathy, the setting aside of social prejudice and patronage for charity's sake. It shows that material help, if these things are lacking, is but as husks, flung before the poor as if they were without common humanity. It is needless to add that religion, if sternly refusing to attract by loaves and fishes, will increase her opportunities for exercising a rightful authority and influence. But committees, it may be said, curtail the proper individuality of the almoner. That is the individual's fault, if it be so. Many work in co-operation, who otherwise would not work at all ; and as inquiry shows the need of that kind of charity which is usually the most neglected, so does the committee afford occasion to each member for meeting, according to the best use of his individual powers, the higher wants of those in trouble or distress. No doubt committees may become official, as individuals may become indolent. Another argument is that people ought only to be asked to state their troubles privately; that, however guarded, their statement is in the nature of a confession, and should be made, heard, and considered in this spirit: the facts ought not to be revealed to more than one or two. Of course such a view is quite inapplicable to scores of the seekers for charity—public opinion in their class has rubbed off this fineness of feeling: it is one of charity's works to replace it. But it is applicable to some cases; and in them the personal and, as it were, private work may well be delegated to an individual, if he be without doubt one who with much kindness of heart is yet sufficiently instructed and experienced to be able to obtain corroborative testimony, and to judge of evidence, for unhappily the stress of life, in which vice plays a part, creates an hypocrisy, the cunning simulation of which has an air of reality, that deceives all but a very few. Next it may be said, true charity recognises no limits; none are so abandoned that it has to give up all hope of their reform. Facts again prove the contrary, with some limitations. When the will is weakened and the nerve irresolute, the lives of many become hopeless: as they have sown they reap; on the bed they have made they lie. Hope must therefore limit its hopefulness; if it be worthy of the name, it must spring from a knowledge of the true condition of the unfortunate, however determined it may be to make the best of the facts. This makes one limit. And there is another. Were all the powers of religious and material charity co-ordinated and available for the rescue of the individual, each ready to assist according to its kind and the circumstances of the patient, the ability of charity to help to good purpose would be enormously increased. As this co-operation becomes a reality, charity will be able to extend its usefulness. Experience, however, of the sum and character of the means available and also of the conditions and causes of distress in a large number of cases, imposes a natural limit to remedial work, which may be gainsaid, but does in the issue prove itself a matter of fact. What that limit is a methodic study of charity and its results will show to each.

These general principles then may be allowed—that charity has to discriminate; that for this and other purposes inquiry is necessary; that, as far as possible, it has to cure and not merely to alleviate distress; that to do this and to know its own limits, it must be instructed in the modes of assisting, spiritual and material; and that to use these modes beneficially the charitable must co-operate—combining the resources of charity, supplementing individual action, and taking common counsel.

VI.—On Interim or Instant Help.

It will be said that while this careful inquiry is being made, and suitable help in all quarters is sought, the applicant will starve; and if the case is ineligible—to be dealt with eventually by the Poor Law—there will be delay none the less, and this delay will be cruel. People in real distress only ask for help, it will be urged, when every other hope has failed; and coming in the direst need, they are quietly left in their need, while elaborate measures are taken to aid them. This evil, so far as it exists, may be met by interim help—especially in cases in which it has been decided to give assistance. The applicant in some instances may be placed in a refuge or other temporary abode. If he has already been in the workhouse, he may be sent to the relieving officer, and the interim help will thus be supplied by the Poor Law, while the case, if suitable, will eventually be helped by charity. The greatest care is necessary in dealing with cases of urgency. Urgency is often the most effective instrument for extorting alms, and many of the poor are quite ready to use it to gain the interim help of a few shillings. They have many resources besides the charity of their superiors. Nothing but a knowledge of their ways of life will be a sufficient guide to the almoner. Yet, as even plausible allegations of hardship are likely to discredit the cause of wise charity, it must be remembered that it is a small matter to spend a few shillings in a case about which you are settling once and for all whether it should be left to the Poor Law or thoroughly dealt with by charity. Were almoners ready to accept some common principles of discrimination, so that ineligible applicants, when adjudicated on, were left to the Poor Law only, instead of having merely one source of charity cut off, interim help might be given and would be fully justified in very many cases. The proper use of the large mass of charity referred to in Section V. of the Register, ' Relief in Distress (temporary),' is for interim help only.

VII.—On Charitable Institutions.

Generally speaking, the test of the usefulness of charitable institutions is, whether or not they produce self-help in the recipients of their bounties and in the people at large. If they do not, they are misnamed charities, for they are undermining the manliness of the people. What then, to prevent their abuse, are the self-imposed safeguards of charities? A consideration of the modes of admission will show that the restrictions have rather the object of limiting their use than of guarding it. Destitution, for instance, is a frequently recurrent condition; but this, so far from being a safeguard, suggests rather a distinction quite unreal from the charitable, as opposed to the Poor Law, point of view, for vice can soon reduce a family to destitution, and improvidence often leaves the individual in extreme want towards the end of life. Charity would rather

The test of charitable institutions.

Restrictions on admission.

prevent destitution, than accept it as a condition of help. Passing by minor restrictions—election by votes is in many large institutions necessary to admission. The evils of this system have been modified in several instances; but it is in principle a limitation and not a safeguard. The chief plea for it is, that large establishments dependent on a regular income must give to each contributor a specific advantage—a *quid pro quo* in the shape of patronage—for otherwise the income would be diminished. The contributor, in fact, purchases by his contribution a quantum of influence in the admission of candidates, according to a regular tariff. The rules of the institution lay down certain conditions, but if these are satisfied, the choice rests with electors, who are canvassed and often induced to subscribe for the benefit of particular candidates. The question therefore is, not which candidate most requires assistance, but which has the most interest: and the fanning up of this interest depends on the circulation of papers and a clever manipulation of the voting power of the institution. A large donor has many votes and much influence. But a large donor has often very little time to learn the relative merits of candidates, and he may be a most uninstructed almoner. As in other matters, the choice demands skill and not a battle of interests. The plea that the system is necessary to the maintenance of institutions is in itself invalid. If the system is working in a manner detrimental to the poor at large it should be altered, or, if the logical alternative must be pressed, it is only right that the institution should be closed. Recent changes and experiments show, however, that it is not necessary to the maintenance of institutions. Admission by election is only one of various similar questions, which ought to be discussed dispassionately and with a recognition of the obvious, but sometimes forgotten, fact that charitable institutions exist only for the benefit of the poor, and have to justify their existence on these terms. No one can pretend to have solved the problem of the best methods of assistance; everyone, therefore, should be ready to make frequent reforms. Charity, by its very nature, is extremely exposed to misuse. Its funds must always be a last hope to indolence and improvidence. Its rules have something of the force of social custom: they re-act on the lives of possible recipients, who form their habits according to the chances open to them. Charity, especially institutional and public charity, must thus, in the interests of the poor, be always in an attitude of wise self-protection, changing and varying its scope and benefits to their needs, and ever working to reduce the number of applicants by initiating them in self-help.

The income of charities. In this book there are entries of Endowed Charities and General Voluntary Charities. Church and Congregational Charities are omitted. It is not possible without a careful analysis of the receipts of these institutions and charities to give any trustworthy estimate of their total income. The total must however be extremely large. An enormous sum is spent annually on begging-letter writers of every kind and degree or given to street mendicants.

The incomes which have been entered in the Register are those returned by the Institutions themselves, but it has not been found possible to compile a satisfactory return of the total income of the charities. Some institutions return their income as 'from all sources,' making no distinction between what is received—*e.g.* from patients and from contributors. Others state their income on one or two heads separately and place the rest of their receipts together, as 'from other sources.' Others return their income under one heading—*e.g.* 'Charitable contributions, bazaars, sales of work,' &c. Others give the gross amount of industrial sales, without deducting the cost of material, labour, &c. Others make a return of income for years, or periods, other than the year last past. A number of institutions make no return whatever as to income. Passing next to the management of institutions, information on this point also has been inserted. It is not enough to have committees, but to have 'working' committees, who understand the accounts and internal arrangements of their institutions or societies. Inquiry not unfrequently proves that the display of names on the cover of a society's report is entirely deceptive. The committee are men of straw; the patrons know nothing of the institution, never make use of it, and support it only by giving their names; the officials are sometimes absolute managers, sometimes even managers primarily in their own interests. Unpaid service, it is said in extenuation, is shifty and irresponsible, but it is well that as many people as possible should be interested in charitable work, even if their services be often only nominal. This argument might be passed by, if the pageantry of names did not cover the working of institutions which are affecting for good or for evil the future lives of many who cannot protest on their own behalf and are practically in the absolute control of their superiors. To guard the donor and the recipient, there ought to be a ready means of ascertaining whether there is a frequent periodical meeting of a committee of management, composed of members qualified to serve from a knowledge of the details of their Society's work and of its general bearing. Charities want not patrons, but workers. They are puffed, advertised, and pleaded for in a self-seeking, self-laudatory style, as if bent on gaining the applause of men ; or they are aided by dinners, festivals, balls, and the like, as if they should find a place among the pastimes of Society and make money out of its fashionable pleasures. Instead of this, they should assume their rightful position

Management of institutions.

as institutions to which in one department the nation entrusts
the constant work of national regeneration.   They would then
combine to put down all that is false in themselves, and expend
and economise their resources in men and money to fulfil this duty
in the most perfect manner.

Next to the constitution of the committee of an institution
come the accounts and the annual report.   A yearly balance-sheet
should be made out and audited by public accountants or other
competent persons, whose addresses should be given.   A report
should be published every year and sent to all subscribers and
donors : to this report should be appended a list of subscribers
and donors, with the amount of their contributions added up and
agreeing with the balance-sheet.

These may seem obvious precautions.   They are, however,
often overlooked.   A friend, who contributes to many institutions,
acts upon and suggests to others the following rules : —

(1) Not to give to charitable institutions that publish no list of contributors.

(2) To require that the amounts in such lists be added up and carried forward from page to page, and finally totalled at the end.'

(3) To pay all contributions by cheque, on account of the charity named,
crossed by its bankers.

In this book *mala fide* charities have been excluded *as far as
possible*: of the comparative utility of those mentioned the reader
must be his own judge.

VIII.—ON DISTRICT VISITING; PERSONAL CHARITY AND WHOLESALE CHARITY.

*Almsgiving
and re-ligious
teaching
should be
separate.*

If the giving of money and tickets is subordinated to the endeavour to influence the poor, personal charity itself, as, for instance, in
visiting the homes of the poor, will assume new conditions.   It is questionable whether ' house-to-house visitation ' is not a waste of energy.
Comparatively few people have the tact and knowledge to be good
District Visitors.   A constant intrusion into the houses of the poor
weakens their self-respect, and, if combined with religious ministra-
tion, tends to hypocrisy.   The tract and the shilling are acceptable,
not the former only.   The dinner or tea before the address is
acceptable, not the latter only.   The separation of religious teaching
and almsgiving is therefore, in the interests of morality, most
necessary.   It will be said, as it is said by many ministers, that,
going to a wretched room, they cannot pray with people who they
think are starving : religious ministrations to people left to famish
seem a cruel mockery.   Yet men, who are intent on doing spiritual
good, whose mood for the time must of necessity be one of hopeful
and intent earnestness, and who are unable for the moment in their
absorption in their object to take notice of details, are quite unfit

then to judge of evidence, and quite liable to deception by those who are callous to their earnestness and in no way scrupulous of acting a part. If this is so, it is best that the question of material assistance should be entrusted to other hands, or at least dealt with at another time. Many cases illustrative of this will be found in Mr. Hornsby Wright's 'Confessions of an Almsgiver,' and 'Thoughts and Experiences of a Charity Organisationist.' Relief will be more wisely granted if it is given apart from religious teaching, and by the direction of a committee, after a discussion of the particulars in each instance.

Instead of 'house-to-house visitation,' a system possible only where the leisurely reside, and therefore inapplicable to the poorest districts, where presumably it should be most required, should be substituted the plan of visiting families in connection with applications for assistance.[1] The appeal for assistance on the applicant's part has given his benefactor a fair opportunity of helping in his own way and on his own conditions. To make inquiries on special points, and for the after-care of the case, when the committee has decided generally on the mode of assisting, personal charity is often required. 'Let the philanthropist be made to understand,' says Chalmers ('On the Sufficiency of the Parochial System'), 'that, for the purpose of doing aught like substantial or permanent good, something more is necessary than to compassionate the poor—he must also consider them ; and let him learn at length that there is indeed a more excellent way of charity than that to which his own headlong sensibilities have impelled him.'

To be competent to visit the poor, the visitor should be able to show them how to economise, how to prepare food simply and well, where to invest savings. She ought to be an authority in domestic business. She ought to know what are the requirements of sanitation. She ought to have that combination of authority and gentleness which wins respect and friendship and can stimulate to duty without giving offence. 'Friendly love perfecteth man.' She should not be an almsgiver, but a friend.

A word may be added here in regard to 'wholesale' charities, such as soup-kitchens and the like. Many of the ordinary parochial charities are planned in the belief that the poor must be expected to receive some sort of charitable assistance every year. Charities, in which, owing to their furnishing the materials, local tradesmen have often an interest, are thus continually checking all tendency towards the establishment of co-operative stores or of any system which

Marginal notes:
The after-care of cases

Qualifications for visitor.

The luxury done by wholesale charity.

---

[1] On this point the reader might find it useful to refer to some of the papers published by the Charity Organisation Society, especially those on 'Volunteer Work.' Much may be said for systematic visitation. If that be preferred, some reasonable pretext for calling is desirable. The collection of rents may serve as this or the weekly collection of savings, or a visit in regard to children who attend a school in which the visitor teaches or is a manager.

may make the poor more independent. Like the villagers who were about to establish a friendly society, but repented when they remembered that for its benefits they would have to pay many annual contributions, and in the end would have no out-relief, while to qualify for out-relief no such contributions were necessary—so the poor may fairly argue that, as relief is both fairly abundant and recurs with the recurrence of the winter, it is against their own interest to make any very hard and unpleasant effort to provide entirely for themselves. If they push themselves out of the class ' poor,' or rather ' indigent,' they lose these casual alms. Indeed, charities given to the multitude are alto-gether wrong. To be beneficial, charity must adjust its means to the wants of the particular case, and not leave that case till it has effected a cure. Wholesale charities either demoralise the poor by their periodicity—*e.g.* in every hard winter—or they feed the casual pauper, who, if charity is plentiful, lives out of the workhouse; or if, as in a mild winter, it is scarce, retires to the more rigorous discipline of the house. The use of the

Charities in kind ; how useful. charities given in kind is limited. They are suitable for interim help until the case is permanently aided ; and they are useful in sick cases, in which nourishing diet is required. The way in which tickets and trifles in food and money are often given is illustrated in the following cases :—

(1) ' This case had long been known to the Committee. The man was a cabman, aged 41, but suffers from gout, and can seldom do any work. The wife applied to a lady in the neighbourhood for assistance. Their rooms were very dirty and untidy, and £3 was due for rent. There were six children, aged from 3 to 21. It was ascertained that the wife and children were earning 28s. a week and some food, and that they were receiving broken food daily from one lady, and 1s. a week from another, and occasional tickets from the clergy, making their income at least 34s. or 35s. a week, besides anything the husband might earn.'

(2) ' A woman and her grown-up daughter, living together, had been receiving charitable tickets for a long time, till the visitor thought it would not be right to spend more on these people, who seemed to get no better off ; and the case was referred to this Committee. On inquiring into particulars it was ascertained that their earnings, though not large, would be sufficient to maintain them, if it was not that their rent was very high— 6s 6d. The Committee persuaded them to move into cheaper lodgings. at 3s. 6d., which were found for them by the Biblewoman ; but to enable them to move, and to prevent their furniture being detained for the heavy arrears of rent they had incurred, about 50s. had to be paid, which was given about half by the rector of the parish and half by the Society for the Relief of Distress. They thus became self-supporting ; but if the tickets had never been given they would have had to move long before ; the 3s. a week which they would thus have saved would have been more to them than the value of the tickets ; and as the arrears of rent would not have been incurred, a little thoughtfulness would both have saved them from being long dependent on charity, and have saved the value of the tickets and the 50s. for more necessitous cases.'

(3) ' A middle-aged single woman, about eight years ago, applied to this Com-mittee. She was represented by all who knew her as highly respectable ; she was said to be well-connected, but she was in great distress, as she could not earn enough to keep herself by needlework. Pending inquiries as to means of permanent employ-ment or assistance, the Committee organised a temporary weekly allowance for

her. But those who gave it were not willing to continue any regular help, the woman herself was not willing to work, unfortunately finding begging easier, and the good connections vanished on inquiry. The Committee then refused further help, unless she took a situation. But other persons took another view of the matter. Whenever she called at certain houses she was sure of "a trifle" in money and food ; from others she would beg for, and receive, 5s. for materials to make up servants' caps, &c., and from many she received help in reply to letters. One lady sent 1s. a week, but inquired no further into her resources. And what was the result ? Side by side with the habit of begging grew the habit of drinking, and last year she was found living in abject wretchedness, in a miserable room containing only a box and a mattress, on bare boards. Still she obtained enough money from "charitable people" to find means to spend her evenings in public-houses, returning intoxicated late in the night. At length her strength held out no longer against such habits, and she found her way to the workhouse, only at first to stay there a short time, and then to come out and drink once more ; but there can be little doubt where her days must end. Her tale is a sad monument to the "cruel kindness" of unthinking charity.'

IX.—THE MUNICIPAL ADMINISTRATION OF THE METROPOLIS.

The local administration of the Metropolis is of so complex a character that attention should be drawn to it at the outset. Here and throughout we wish to place before the reader the charities on the one hand, and on the other the legislative provisions for the relief of affliction and destitution.

The area of the Metropolis is different, and differently divided, for different purposes. The most important area of administration is that known as 'the Metropolitan area.' It covers 75,462 acres, and in 1891 it contained a population of 4,211,743. It now forms the new county of London (*see* p. cl.). (1) For the election of members of Parliament it is divided into 58 boroughs and electoral divisions, each of which returns one member, excepting the City, which returns two. For the election of members of the County Council the same electoral districts are used. The registered 'County electors' elect 118 members, two for each division, excepting the City, which has four. (2) For the purposes of local management, local drainage, sanitation, etc., the Metropolitan area is divided into 27 parishes, each under a Vestry elected by the parochial electors, and 13 District Boards of Works, including the Woolwich Local Board (*see* p. cxlviii.). (3) For the administration of the Poor Law there are, in the Metropolitan area, 30 Poor Law parishes or unions. In each of these there is a Board of Guardians elected by the parochial electors (*see* p. xxiv.), and entrusted with the legal relief of the poor.[1] (5) For the management of Asylums for Imbeciles and Idiots (*see* p. cxxxviii.), and of Hospitals for

[1] In the Metropolis for Poor Law purposes there are 14 parishes and 16 unions. For brevity's sake, however, the word 'Union' has been generally used (*see also* p. xlvii.). A Union is a union of two or more parishes, each of which send its representatives to a common Board of Guardians. The parish (29 & 30 Vict., c. 1 3, s. 18, and the Interpretation Act 1889) is a place for which a separate poor-rate is, or can be, made, or for which a separate overseer is, or can be, appointed.

Infectious Diseases (see p. cxli.), there is a Metropolitan Asylums Board, consisting of representatives of the Poor Law parishes and unions, and members nominated by the Local Government Board (see p. cxxxiii.). (6) For the administration of the School Board, and for the election of its members, the Metropolitan area is divided into 11 parts (see p. cvii.). The members of the Board are elected by the ratepayers, except in the City, where the voters include all the Parliamentary voters. (7) There is the Police. The Metropolitan Police District covers the area within a radius of 15 miles from Charing Cross. The City has an independent administration of police. (8) For magisterial purposes, the Metropolis is divided into 13 Police Court districts, in addition to two courts held in the City. The Metropolitan police courts are named from the streets or districts where they are held—Bow Street, Westminster, Marlborough Street, Marylebone, Clerkenwell, Thames, Southwark, Lambeth, Worship Street, Dalston (or North London), Hammersmith, Wandsworth (or South-Western), and Greenwich with Woolwich. Except at the last-named courts, which are open, the former from 10 a.m. to 1.30, and the latter from 2.30 p.m. to 5, a magistrate is in attendance daily from 10 to 5. The City police courts are at the Justice Rooms in the Mansion House and the Guildhall. They are open daily from 10 to 4, and on Saturdays from 10 to 1. (9) The Metropolis is divided into the districts (generally conterminous with the parishes or unions) and sub-districts of the Registrar-General for statistical purposes, returns of births and deaths, etc. (10) The local government of the City is in the hands of a Court of Common Council consisting of 26 Aldermen, out of whom the Lord Mayor is annually elected,[1] and 206 Common Councillors. Both Aldermen and Common Councillors are elected by the Parliamentary voters in the City,[2] the former for life, the latter annually. The elections are by wards, of which there are 26. The duties which elsewhere devolve upon a Vestry or District Board are there entrusted to Commissioners of the Sewers, appointed by the Court of Common Council. It is almost inevitable that an almoner should be brought into contact with most of these bodies, or have to ascertain their duties on some points, in order to endeavour to remove evils and to assist cases which he will meet with in the course of his work.

---

[1] The City Livery Companies have an indirect influence on the government of the City. There are 74 of these Companies. Their 'Liverymen' form the chief part of the Court of Common Hall of the City of London. This Court of Common Hall consists of 'the Lord Mayor, at least four Aldermen, and such of the Liverymen of the various City Companies as are of one year's standing, free of the City, and have paid their livery fees.' It elects the City Sheriffs, Chamberlain, Bridge Masters, and Auditors. The Lord Mayor is elected from amongst such of the Aldermen as have served as City Sheriff.—See 'Greater London and its Government,' by George Whale, and Firth's 'Municipal London.'

[2] The 'Liverymen, free by birth or servitude, and residing within twenty-five miles of the City,' are among the Parliamentary voters in the City.

X.—On the Functions of the Poor Law and of Charity.

It has been said above that charity, as there is a Poor Law in England, may safely restrict itself to eligible cases. It is hardly too much to say that no person should take part in at least public charitable work without a general knowledge of the functions of the Poor Law.

The claim for Poor Law relief rests, it may be broadly stated, upon the destitution of the claimant. Merit has nothing to do with it. The vicious and virtuous are equally entitled to it. The humane from motives of charity, and the prosperous from motives of self-protection, would not suffer the destitute to starve. A Poor Law was therefore established. But neither would they tempt the self-supporting to destitution. Therefore it was established under just but hard restrictions. 'The fundamental principle '—to quote the often-quoted passage of the report of the Poor Law Commissioners, 1834—' with respect to the legal relief of the poor is, that the condition of the pauper ought to be on the whole less eligible than that of the independent labourer. The equity and expediency of this principle are equally obvious. Unless the condition of the pauper is on the whole less eligible than that of the independent labourer, the law destroys the strongest motives to good conduct, steady industry, providence, and frugality among the labouring classes, and induces persons, by idleness or imposture, to throw themselves upon the poor rates for support.' The independent labourer has to be protected only against destitution. 'The pauper has no just ground for complaint, if at the same time that his physical wants are amply provided for, his condition should be less eligible than that of the poorest class of those who contribute to his support.'[1] On the threshold of the question then we see the boundary lines of charity and the Poor Law. To charity it is not a matter of primary importance, whether a person is destitute or not. For it destitution is no test. It has more chance of helping effectually if a person be not destitute. It has to prevent destitution and indigence. It may have to supply actual necessaries, but to place the poor beyond the reach of need or to prevent the recurrence of need is its true vocation. It is unlimited in its scope, and gives as a free gift. From the point of view of the Poor Law the question of destitution is all-important. It is the passport to relief. Its

The main difference between Poor Law relief and Charitable relief.

---

[1] Subject to modifications, to be subsequently mentioned, but which do not materially affect the general principle—' The function of the Guardians is to relieve destitution actually existing, and not to expend the money of the ratepayers in preventing a person becoming destitute, that is to say, they can only expend the poor rates in supplying the destitute persons with actual necessaries, such as food, clothing, or lodging, or the means of obtaining food, clothing, or lodging temporarily, if the destitute person cannot be immediately received into the workhouse.'—' The Poor Law Orders of the Poor Law Commissioners, the Poor Law Board, and the Local Government Board,' by W. Cunningham Glen, 1883 p 63,

administration is tied and bound with restrictions. Its supplies are
drawn from a ratepayers' trust fund. Its main purpose is not
to prevent or remove distress, but to alleviate it. It is a stern
alleviative measure. It helps only when it must; charity always
when it wills. Charity like the Poor Law may destroy 'the
strongest motives to good conduct, steady industry, providence, and
frugality.' Investigation, fortified by tests, guards the one; knowledge and inquiry ought to guard the other.

XI.—THE ADMINISTRATION OF THE POOR LAWS: THE LOCAL GOVERNMENT BOARD.

The administration of Poor Law relief is vested in the Board of
Guardians, the local authority established for the purpose in each
union, subject to the direction and control of the Local Government
Board, the central authority. The Board by elaborate 'orders' and
numerous forms has settled with precision the duties of each officer
to be employed by the Guardians, how their establishments are to
be managed, how their accounts are to be kept, and generally how
their relief is to be given.[1] Without the consent of the Local
Government Board the Guardians may neither appoint nor remove
any officer. On the other hand, the limitations to the powers of the
Local Government Board are these: it cannot interfere with the
laws of settlement and removal (of which a few words further on);
it cannot order relief in a particular case; and it cannot compel
attendance at a worship, or education in a religious creed, objected
to by the pauper.

The Local Government Board (Whitehall) is composed of a
President (at present the Right Hon. G. Shaw-Lefevre, M.P.), and
as *ex-officio* members, the Lord President of the Privy Council, the
principal Secretaries of State, the Lord Privy Seal and the
Chancellor of the Exchequer. For the supervision of the local administration the Board has Inspectors and Auditors. The former are
entitled to visit workhouses, attend and, without a vote, take part in
meetings of Boards of Guardians, and to hold inquiries and summon
witnesses in regard to any question of Poor Law administration.
The latter have full powers to 'examine, audit, allow or disallow
of accounts and of items therein.' Any payment at variance
with the rules or orders of the Local Government Board is dis-
allowed, though the Board has discretionary power of remitting
the disallowance surcharged. There is thus a very strict control.

---

[1] ' As regards the relief of persons who are in receipt of charitable contributions, it may be observed that if the fact comes to the knowledge of the Guardians,
in the case of an application to them for relief, they are bound to act upon it, and
either wholly refuse relief, or to give such an amount only as, with the other
assistance the applicant receives, will be sufficient to relieve his actual necessities.'
Glen · Poor Law Orders. p. 64 (1883).

In the Metropolitan area there are three Inspectors and two Auditors, and there are 30 Parishes or Unions.

XII.—The Board of Guardians: Illustrations of the Importance of Co-operation with the Charitable.

The population and area of these Unions is stated in the local lists (printed in the Register), with the addresses of the District Schools, Workhouses, Casual wards, and other particulars.

If there is thorough co-operation between the Guardians and charitable persons on sound principles, many cases of distress which would otherwise have been improperly or insufficiently assisted, will be carefully attended to. Two plans of co-operation may be mentioned. At Kensington members of the Charity Organisation Committee see most of the applicants for out-relief, and at once interfere if they think their money or advice can prevent a man from becoming a pauper. Similarly, they and other charitable persons are constantly examining the more hopeful of the inmates of the workhouse, and are ready to do what they can to restore the paupers to independence. In order to investigate these cases more closely, members of the Charity Organisation Committee attend the meetings of the Guardians' House Committee, and a Sub-Committee of the Charity Organisation Committee meets at the workhouse. The following instances show how such plans of co-operation work :—

Evidence of the advantage of co-operation between Poor Law and Charity.

A., a young woman, presented herself for admission to the workhouse, but the officer who saw her, struck by her appearance and manner, advised her, before taking any further step, to consult a lady, a member of this Committee, whose address he gave her. She did so, and, her story being at once inquired into, it appeared that she had been in highly respectable service; had left to nurse a sister in ill-health, on whom she spent all her savings; had come to London on her sister's death, hoping to find employment, but failed ; and, finding herself getting into debt, had resolved, in desperation, to seek refuge in the workhouse. Assistance was immediately given her, the money necessary to get requisite clothing was advanced, and employment obtained for her. She is now in a superior situation, has repaid the money lent to her, and acknowledged with deep gratitude the help which saved her.

B., a girl of wandering habits, but apparently not of bad character, who had drifted into the workhouse, was sent to a training home and thence to service.

A widow of 47, who was in receipt of parish relief, asked for help. She had four daughters of earning age. The home was very dirty, and the family of low type. The Committee decided not to assist the family with money, but advised the mother to try and get work, and offered to assist in improving the position of any of the daughters. The second one, a cripple of no occupation, was the only one who consented to be helped. Medical opinion was taken, and a boot supplied her at a cost of 23s. The boot was found to be of very little, if any, use, and the girl was sent to the Westminster Hospital. It was decided that an operation was necessary. This was done, and later on a second one, and the doctor ordered a surgical appliance, which was supplied by the Committee at a cost of £3. 10s. The girl was sent to a home (where she improved very much) to learn housework, and afterwards a situation was found for her. This she lost at once through temper. Another situation was found her, where she seemed comfortably settled, and was left to the care of the Metropolitan Association for Befriending Young Servants.

H. T. This old man was referred to the Committee by a member of the Board of Guardians. T. is aged 77. His wife is 74, and paralysed. He has worked 30 years for one firm, he has been 30 years in a friendly society, which he helped to found, and he has been for 50 years a member of his trade society. His friendly society has no superannuation allowance. His only child, a daughter, is married to a brushmaker, and she keeps a sweet shop. She helps her old parents as far as she can, and, living in the immediate neighbourhood, sends one of her children to look after them. T. is in receipt of 6s. a week from his trade society, and this Committee have raised a pension of 5s. a week for him. In the middle of next year he will receive from his friendly society 8s. a week for 12 weeks, and after that 4s. a week for 12 weeks. The Committee will regulate their pension accordingly.

In the following case, in which defects of character had brought the applicant to the workhouse, it was found impossible to rescue him. 'L.' a painter, was given a fresh start after being many months in the workhouse. He did a good summer's work, earning from 30s. to £2 a week, but he afterwards applied again to the Guardians for relief, and probably spent the winter with his family in the workhouse.

At Kensington a Workhouse Girls' Aid Committee has also been formed. A member of the Committee takes down the case of each girl. Inquiries are made either by the Charity Organisation Society or by a lady familiar with their practice. If the Committee are satisfied that the girl wishes to lead a better life, a situation is looked out for her, and help granted according to her requirements for herself and for her child. Parents are sought out. Mother and child are visited periodically, and payments received on the children's behalf. At St. Pancras and elsewhere there are similar committees.

There are thus many reasons why those who possess time and leisure, and desire to undertake charitable work, should become members of Boards of Guardians.

XIII.—The Election of Boards of Guardians: its Importance.

The Local Government Act 1894.

The Local Government Act of 1894 has placed the election of Poor Law Guardians and, subject to the orders of the Local Government Board, the whole management of the Poor Law, in the hands of the parochial electors. Whatever it may have been in the past, now at least in one sense the administration of the Poor Law will be popular. In future there will be no plural vote, no necessary qualification by rate, no *ex-officio* Guardians : the elections will be by ballot ; and any resident of twelve months may stand for election. Now, therefore, it is the task of the true reformer to make the Poor Law popular in the best sense of the word. It should not, under its new administrators, become an institution which the people will regard as a mere source of relief, distributed according to the seeming wants of particular cases, but it should be a system of relief administered with justice, and in such a way that those who, from feebleness of character, poorness of spirit, or carelessness easily slip into habits of dependence, shall not be tempted to rely on any help except the help of their own heads and hands. These principles are quite compatible with a thoughtful and kindly provision for the sick and also for the aged, for whose maintenance no other and better source of assistance is available; but they may quickly be forgotten, and the country may become involved in many old evils, habited in new guises and called by new names, if the administration of the Poor Law is not as deliberative, conscientious, and even, as in the last twenty years it has tended to become. If on the old system it was the duty of those who enjoyed the magnified influence of the plural vote to take part in Poor Law elections, now they should do more. They should explain their views fully and support them by appeals to personal and general experience; and they should show that good sense, kindness, and real humanity form the groundwork of methods of relief which at first sight may appear to many over-precise and unsympathetic. Mistakes may now very likely be made, with the result that pauperism will increase; but, unless the whole policy of electing the Poor Law Guardians by popular vote is a vast and irreparable mistake, we must believe that the change will produce good and not evil, and that the new electorate will be open to persuasion and guidance, if men and women of the same earnestness and ability as those who have in the last generation devoted themselves to this branch of work, come forward and use their influence wisely and persistently. Then the spirit of opposition to the Poor Law which often shows itself, and which is now used sometimes as a political lever, will be superseded by a spirit of confidence. It will no longer be felt to be a harsh system devised and controlled to protect the pockets of the richer ratepayers, and to dole out meagre relief to the indigent, but a system administered equitably for the well-being of the community as a whole, by the representatives of the whole people.

There are two main points to be explained : (I.) What is the new franchise for election on Boards of Guardians ; (II.) Who are qualified to serve as candidates. We have also (III.) to touch on a few miscellaneous points of importance.

I. The change that has taken place may be summed up in two words : the parochial elector has taken the place of the ratepayer. But some preliminary explanation is needed. *The parochial elector.*

Before the Local Government Act of 1894 [1] was passed the country, apart from other administrative districts not important for our purpose, was divided into Parishes—places where 'a separate poor rate is, or can be, made,' or for which 'a separate overseer is, or can be, appointed' [2]—Rural and Urban Sanitary Districts, Unions of Parishes for Poor Law purposes, Municipal and County Boroughs, and Counties. The Local Government Act of 1888 reformed the

---

[1] Local Government Act 1894, 56 & 57 Vict., c. 73.
[2] The Interpretation Act 1889, 52 & 53 Vict., c. 63, s. 4.

administration of the larger areas, the Counties. The Act of 1894 reformed that of the lesser areas, some for the purposes of general administration, all for the purposes of the Poor Law. In future therefore :—

1. Each Rural Parish will have a Parish Meeting or Parish Council.[1]

2. Each Rural or Urban Sanitary District will have its District Council.

3. As the Rural Parishes before elected Guardians, who were also the Rural Sanitary Authority, so now they will elect District Councillors who will represent the parish as (a) District Councillors, and (b) Guardians, and as Guardians they will be an administrative body separate and distinct from the District Council.

4. Elsewhere—i.e. everywhere except in Rural Districts—there will be Boards of Guardians as heretofore.

5. When the Union includes part of a Rural and part of an Urban District, the Rural Parishes within it will send their Councillors to the Board of Guardians, the Urban Parishes their Guardians.

6. But everywhere the members of Boards of Guardians will, like Rural or Urban District Councillors, be elected by the parochial electors.

7. To be a parochial elector a person must have his or her name on the Local Government register of electors, or the Parliamentary register of electors, so far as they relate to the parish. These two registers together form the register of the parochial electors.[2]

The names on these registers make up a constituency of every rank and class.

A.—THE PARLIAMENTARY REGISTER.

The Register of Parochial Electors. Subject to disqualifications to be mentioned below, the following qualifications entitle a man of full age to have his name placed on this register :—

1. As OWNER: if he is the owner of—

(a) A freehold of forty shillings clear yearly value if the estate be for inheritance, or in actual occupation, or acquired by marriage settlement, devise, or promotion to any benefice or office ;

(b) A freehold of five pounds clear yearly value if an estate for life or lives ;

(c) A copyhold or other tenure (not freehold) held for lives, or any larger estate, of the clear yearly value of five pounds ;

(d) A leasehold of five pounds clear yearly value if originally created for a period of not less than sixty years, or of not less than fifty pounds clear yearly value if originally created for a term of not less than twenty years.

2. As to OCCUPATION: the following have the franchise as occupiers :—

(a) Every man of full age, who is the occupier (whether owner or tenant) and for twelve months previous to the fifteenth of July has been the occupier, of lands or tenements in the parish of the value of ten pounds, the rates on which have been paid ;

[1] Where the Urban Sanitary Authority was the Corporation or Council of a Borough, that title remains. Vestries in the Metropolis retain their title (see p. cxlix.).

[2] Local Government Act 1894, s. 44.

(b) Every inhabitant male of full age, who has on the fifteenth of July and during the whole of the preceding twelve months occupied, as owner or tenant, or by virtue of any office or service, a dwelling-house, or any part of a dwelling-house, which has been rated and on which the rates have been paid;

(c) Every occupier of lodgings, being a man of full age, of the clear yearly value unfurnished of ten pounds, who has resided in them for the whole of twelve months previously to the fifteenth of July of the year in which he claims to be registered.

B.—The Local Government (or County) Register.

To be qualified as an elector on this register, it is necessary (1) to be registered as a county elector; and (2) to be entitled to register under the County Electors Act 1888 (sections 2 and 3).[1] There are two franchises: the extended burgess franchise, and the ten pounds occupation qualification. Under the former a person is not entitled to be registered unless qualified as follows : -

Qualification of electors. (1) The extended burgess franchise.

(a) Is of full age on or before the preceding fifteenth of July;

(b) Is on the fifteenth of July in any year, and has been during the whole of the then last preceding twelve months, in occupation, joint or several, of any house, warehouse, counting-house, shop, or other building (in this Act referred to as qualifying property) in the county; and

(c) Has during the whole of those twelve months resided in the county or within fifteen miles thereof;[2] and

(d) Has been rated in respect of the qualifying property to all poor rates made during those twelve months for the parish wherein the property is situate; and

(e) Has on or before the twentieth of the same July paid all such rates, including county rates (if any), as have become payable by him in respect of the qualifying property up to the then last preceding fifth of January.[3]

Under the ten pounds qualification franchise a person is not entitled to be registered unless qualified as follows :—

(2) The ten pounds occupation qualification.

(a) He must, during the whole twelve months immediately preceding the fifteenth day of July, have been an occupier as owner or tenant of some land or tenement in the county of the clear yearly value of not less than ten pounds; and

(b) Must have resided in or within fifteen miles of the county during six months immediately preceding the fifteenth day of July; and

(c) Such person, or some one else, must, during the said twelve months, have been rated to all poor rates made in respect of such land or tenement; and

(d) All sums due in respect of the said land or tenement on account of any poor rate made and allowed during the twelve months immediately preceding the fifth of January next before the registration, or on account of any assessed taxes due before the said fifth day of January, must have been paid on or before the twentieth day of July.

---

[1] *See* the 'County Councillor's Guide,' pp. 253, 254, 195, 203.

[2] 'The name of the person must appear in the rate book, and an occupier who pays or tenders to the overseers the amount due for his poor rate is entitled to have his name registered, and, even if the overseers fail to enrol it, he is nevertheless deemed to be rated. Where a person succeeds to property by descent, marriage, marriage settlement, devise, or promotion to a benefice or office, the occupancy and rating of his predecessor are equivalent to those of his successor.'

[3] When the owner pays the poor rate, there is by the Poor Rate Assessment and Collection Act a constructive payment by the occupier.

Joint occupiers, if the value of the land or tenement is such as to give £10 or more to each occupier, are entitled to register.

Every person (including unmarried women and widows, of full age) so qualified shall be entitled to be registered as a London county elector, unless he be (a) an alien, or (b) has, within the twelve months aforesaid, received union or parochial relief or other alms; or (c) is disentitled under any Act of Parliament, e.g. convicted of treason or felony or of corrupt practices at elections. A person in receipt of parochial relief is thus under (b) disentitled, but with the following exceptions: if parochial relief is given to his blind or deaf and dumb wife, child, or children; if such relief is given to his father; if he accepts public vaccination; if the Guardians pay his children's fees; if he receive assistance by admission to a hospital of the Metropolitan Asylums Board (52 & 53 Vict., c. 56, s. 3), or by the receipt 'for himself or any of his family, of any medical or surgical assistance or any medicine at the expense of any poor rate.' Medical and surgical assistance is defined as including 'all medical and surgical attendance, and all matters and things supplied by or on the recommendation of the medical officer having authority to give such attendance and recommendation at the expense of the poor rate' (48 & 49 Vict., c. 46). Further, a person is not disentitled to be registered (Municipal Corporations Act 1882, 45 & 46 Vict., c. 50, s. 33) if he has received medical and surgical assistance from the trustees of the county charities, or has been removed, by order of a justice, to a hospital or place of reception for the sick at the cost of any local authority; nor if his child has been admitted to and taught in any public or endowed school.[1]

If a person's name is on the register of parochial electors, that is in itself sufficient evidence that he has the right to vote.[2]

The Women's Vote. Finally, not only unmarried women and widows are entitled to vote, but married women also, if they are qualified; that is, if they possess any of the qualifications required for registration in the Local Government register. A husband and wife cannot be qualified in respect of the same property,[3] but if, for instance, one is entered as owner and the other as occupier of different properties in the same parish, each may vote for that parish.

---

[1] Cf. 'London Government,' pp. 236 and 248. It would seem that where, as in Rural Districts, the work of the Poor Law Guardians will, under the Local Government Act of 1894, be placed in the hands of District Councillors, those who receive medical relief as defined by 48 & 49 Vict. c. 46, the Medical Relief Disqualification Act, will retain their franchise, although in voting for District Councillors they will also be voting for Guardians. But in Urban Districts, where the Boards of Guardians still remain separate bodies, they will be able to vote (as in London) for the Local Board or Vestry, but not for the Board of Guardians.

[2] Local Government Act 1894, s. 44 (1).

[3] Sec. 43.

These paragraphs on the parochial electorate may seem rather intricate, and after all reference must be often had to technical books when questions of difficulty arise. But it is worth while to study with some closeness the question who is a parochial elector, when so much turns upon local elections.

II. 'Next, in regard to the qualification of candidates: A person shall not be qualified to be elected or to be a Guardian for a Poor Law Union unless' (according to the Local Goverment Act 1894)— *Local Government Act 1894, c. 73, s. 20 (2).*

'(1) He is a parochial elector; or

'(2) Has during the whole of the twelve months preceding the election resided in the Union, or

'(3) [Unless] in the case of a Guardian for a parish wholly or partly situate within the area of a borough, whether a county borough or not, he is qualified to be elected a councillor for that borough;

'And no person shall be disqualified by sex or marriage for being elected or being a Guardian.'

Therefore all persons, men or women, are eligible for service as Guardians who are either (1) parochial electors, or (2) twelve months' residents. The candidates may thus be chosen from an even wider field than the electorate.

III. Lastly, some miscellaneous points.

(1) Nominations must be made in writing on papers provided by the returning officer, usually the Clerk to the Guardians. The nomination paper must be signed 'by two parochial electors of the parish or other area as proposer and seconder, and no more, and shall state their respective places of abode.' The parochial elector can only sign a nomination paper for any parish or other area for which he is registered as a parochial elector; and he can sign papers for only one parish or other area. He cannot nominate a larger number of candidates than the total number that are to be elected for that parish or area.

(2) 'Each elector may give one vote and no more for each of any number of persons not exceeding the number to be elected.' [2]

(3) The poll on the day of election must be open between 6 and 8 in the evening.

(4) The term of office of a Guardian is three years, but 'one-third, as nearly as may be, of every Board of Guardians shall go out of office on the fifteenth day of April in each year, and their places shall be filled by the newly-elected Guardians.' A County Council is, however, empowered, on application from a Board of Guardians, to order a retirement of the whole Board every third year.

---

[1] '"Residence" appears to mean a personal dwelling within the union, as distinguished from the mere occupation of property. For some purposes a person may have more than one residence. Thus he may have houses in different places, each of which may be called his residence; but it may be doubted whether, for purposes of this Act, a man can reside in more than one place.' *See* The Local Government Act 1894, p. 122. Macmorran & Dill.

[2] Sec. 20 (4).

(5) 'A Board of Guardians may elect a chairman or vice-chairman, or both, and not more than two other persons from outside their own body, but from persons qualified to be Guardians of the Union, and any person so elected shall be an additional Guardian and member of the Board.'

It is greatly hoped that readers of this 'Introduction' will take an active interest in the election of Guardians wherever they may have votes, and, if they are almoners, wherever their work may lie. A misguided or lavish bestowal of Poor Law relief produces evil results on character and on family life with which the most widely diffused State education cannot cope. The Board of Guardians are in the most practical, forcible manner — viz. by giving or withholding relief—either the moral instructors or the well-intentioned enemies of that large section of the poor which is on the verge of pauperism.

XIV.—THE DUTIES OF GUARDIANS IN REGARD TO INDOOR AND OUTDOOR RELIEF.

Under the management of the Guardians are Workhouses, Infirmaries, and Schools (Indoor Relief) ; Casual wards and casual relief; and outdoor general and medical relief, including medical relief at Poor Law Dispensaries. In the Metropolis several unions share District Schools and other establishments. What these are will be seen in the local lists.

Workhouse cases.

The workhouse (or rather, perhaps, we should say, indoor relief) is the corner-stone of the English Poor Law system. That combination of buildings which is usually called the 'workhouse,' consists of wards or blocks for old men, for old women, for able-bodied men, and for able-bodied women, and for children also, if they are not lodged in a separate or district school. It has a nursery. It affords shelter to persons of unsound or feeble mind and epileptics. It has sick wards or an infirmary. And it has a casual ward. It is an institution partly alleviative, partly restrictive. It is alleviative because it is intended to supply nothing beyond humane and considerate relief, including, of course, curative relief to the sick, and depauperising education to the children. It is restrictive because it is managed in such a way as not to attract claimants, but to limit relief to those who cannot maintain themselves. The cases which charity may fitly leave to the Guardians for indoor treatment are incurable cases of vice and intemperance ; chronic cases, i.e. cases of intermittent need, in which no provision is or can be made for future contingencies; or cases of continuous need, in which, owing to the applicant's fault, no provision has been made for old age, and in which without an allowance he will lack the means of subsistence; cases in which relatives are able to assist adequately, and avoid doing so ; able-bodied persons out of work and with no definite prospect of work.

This list does not pretend to be exhaustive; and it is charity's first duty to take each case on its merits. An off-hand classification of charitable applications as falling under any of the above categories is greatly to be deprecated. But here we have only to consider in some detail what the distinctions are which the Guardians themselves have to draw between indoor and outdoor relief, and what are the arrangements of a workhouse.

A pauper is defined as any ' person maintained wholly or in part A pauper. by or chargeable to any parish, borough, or city.'[1] But a person who receives medical or surgical assistance, or any medicine at the expense of any poor rate for himself or any of his family, is not a pauper, in the sense that he does not lose his vote for Parliamentary and County Council elections. He has, however, no vote for the election of Guardians.[2] Also, elementary education of a blind or deaf and dumb child does not deprive the parent of any franchise[3]; and there are other exceptions (see p. xxviii.).

In the Returns published by the Local Government Board, the 'indoor paupers' include the paupers in all the establishments under the control of the Guardians, and also in some establishments not under their management, such as certified schools, schools for deaf, blind, and idiots.[4] Children boarded-out are entered as in receipt of outdoor relief. The classes of paupers, in and outdoor, are the able-bodied male and female, and their children under 16; the not able-bodied male and female, and their children, or children without parents; the insane and idiots, and vagrants. Another sub-division has also been introduced recently. The able-bodied indoor paupers are divided, both males and females, into the two categories, 'In health,' and 'Temporarily disabled.' The able-bodied out-door male paupers are also divided into two classes: ' Relieved on account of their own sickness, accident, or infirmity,' and ' Relieved from other causes.' By this means the pauperism due to sickness may in some degree be discriminated from the pauperism due to other causes.[5]

For the guidance of Guardians in the administration of outdoor relief there are three Orders. Firstly, the General Prohibitory Order (Dec. 21, 1844). This applies to the larger number of Unions, but not to Unions in the Metropolis, or to Manchester, Liverpool, Newcastle-on-Tyne, and several other large towns. It

[1] See Glen, p. 192.
[2] Medical Relief Disqualification Removal Act 1885 (48 & 49 Vict., c. 46). See ante, page xxviii., and Note.
[3] Elementary Education (Blind and Deaf Children) Act 1893, 56 & 57 Vict., c. 42, s. 10. See also pp. cxxix. and cxxxi.
[4] See Local Government Report 1887-8, pp. 187, 188.
[5] In compiling the statistical portion of the Outdoor Relief List, the following rules are observed. If the relief is granted to the head of the family for himself [or herself], then he and all the family dependent on him are entered as relieved. If the relief is granted to the head of the family for a member or members of his family, then the number of members relieved is entered plus one for the head of the family. See Poor Law General Orders (Macmorran and Lushington, p. 417).

indicates the high-water mark of the actual prohibition of outdoor relief at the present time. Next, there is the Outdoor Labour Test Order (Oct. 31, 1842). This applies to many of the Unions under the Prohibitory Order, and may be considered as an appendix to it. Thirdly, there is the Outdoor Relief Regulation Order (Dec. 14, 1852), which applies to the Metropolis and the larger towns.

Several of the more advanced metropolitan Boards of Guardians are now in practice adopting an administration of outdoor relief in accordance with the Prohibitory Order. They are making the grant of out-relief the exception instead of the rule. It is desirable, therefore, to place an outline of both Orders before the reader.

The Prohibitory Order: Residents. The Prohibitory Order falls into two main sections: relief to cases resident in the Union; relief to non-resident cases.

Subject to certain exceptions mentioned below, in cases resident in the Union, relief, except in the workhouse, is prohibited to any able-bodied person, male or female, or to such members of his or her family ' as may reside with him or her, and may not be in employment,' or to the wife of such able-bodied person, if she be resident with him.

Whether a person is or is not able-bodied is a question of fact depending upon the physical strength and condition of the applicant for relief. Thus, children of 14 or 15, able to maintain themselves, may be considered able-bodied, and a man over 60 is not necessarily ' not able-bodied.' [1]

The exceptions then follow :

Relief out of the workhouse is not prohibited to an able-bodied person, where such person

(1) Shall require relief on account of sudden or urgent necessity ;

(2) Shall require relief on account of any sickness, accident, or bodily or mental infirmity affecting such person, or any of his or her family ;

(3) Shall require relief for the purpose of defraying the expenses, either wholly or in part, of the burial of his or her family ;

(4) Shall require relief, being a widow in the first six months of widowhood ;

(5) Shall require relief, being a widow, who has a legitimate child or children dependent on her, is incapable of earning his, her, or their livelihood, and has no illegitimate children born after the commencement of her widowhood ;

(6) Shall require relief, being a wife, whose husband is confined in any gaol or place of safe custody (subject to Article 4, quoted below) [1]

(7) Shall be the wife or child of any able-bodied man who shall be in the service of Her Majesty, as a soldier, sailor, or marine.

[1] See Glen. pp. 422, 414 (ed. 1883).

(8) 'Where any able-bodied person, not being a soldier, sailor, or marine, shall not reside within the Union, but his wife, child, or children shall reside within the same, the Board of Guardians of the Union, according to their discretion, may (subject to the regulation contained in Article 4) afford relief in the workhouse to such wife, child, or children, or may allow outdoor relief for any such child or children being within the age of nurture [*i.e.* seven years old], and resident with the mother within the Union.'

The Article 4 of the Order referred to above in exceptions (6) and (8) is as follows:—

'Where a husband of any woman is beyond the seas [*i.e.* out of Great Britain], or in custody of the law, or in confinement in a licensed house or asylum as a lunatic or idiot, all relief which the Guardians shall give to the wife, or her child or children, shall be given to such woman in the same manner, and subject to the same conditions, as if she were a widow.'

The conclusions to be drawn from the exceptions (6) and (8) and the Article 4, appear to be, that 'able-bodied women deserted by their husbands should only receive relief in the workhouse'; but 'if such a woman requires relief for her children, any child under the age of nurture and residing with the mother may receive outdoor relief, but the children above that age must be taken into the workhouse.' If, however, the husband has gone beyond the seas, is in gaol, or confined as a lunatic, she is entitled to relief as if she were a widow.

To non-residents the Order prohibits outdoor relief, except in the workhouse, unless (1) where such person, being casually within such parish, shall become destitute. The Prohibitory Order. Non-residents.

This covers relief to vagrants; as to the provision for whom *see* p. lix.

Or (2), where such person shall require relief on account of any sickness, accident, or bodily or mental infirmity affecting such person or any of his or her family.

Then follow other exceptions to the prohibition, two of which may be noted: an exception by which outdoor relief may be given to a widow not resident in the Union for the first six months of widowhood; and an exception by which such relief may be given to a widow who has a legitimate child or children dependent on her (*see* above (5)), and who at the time of her husband's death was resident with him in some other place than the parish of her legal settlement, and not situated in the Union in which such parish may be comprised. The object of this clause 'appears to be to avoid the disturbance of those connections and mode of life at a distance from the Union to which the family may have become accustomed, and which existed at the time of the husband's death.'

The Prohibitory Order, it will be noticed, prohibits and regulates relief in the case of able-bodied men and women only. It neither prohibits nor regulates relief to those who are not able-bodied. Hence it in no way interferes with or alters that part of the law of Queen Elizabeth which provides for 'the necessary relief of the lame, impotent, old, blind, and such other among them being poor and not able to work.' In all these cases the Guardians can provide 'necessary' indoor or outdoor relief as they may think best.

The Outdoor Test Regulation Order, as has been said, supplements the Prohibitory Order. It requires the Guardians, if they depart from the instructions in regard to able-bodied paupers, and relieve them out of the workhouse, (1) to give half of the relief in food, clothing, and other articles of necessity; (2) to give no relief while the able-bodied person is employed for wages or hire or remuneration by any person; (3) to set every such pauper to work;[1] (4) to report to the Local Government Board within fourteen days from the date when this Order comes into force, and from time to time afterwards, as to the place of work, kind of work, &c.

The Outdoor Relief Regulation Order (that applicable to the Metropolis) may be divided into three chief sections; dealing with resident cases, with non-resident cases, and with the employment of the able-bodied. It is limited to setting forth certain conditions under which outdoor relief shall be given; but the general view of the Board is as follows :—

'The Board' (as the letter of instruction to Boards of Guardians in regard to this Order states), 'are of opinion that where there is a commodious and efficient workhouse, it is best that the able-bodied pauper should be received and set to work therein; but looking to the circumstances of most unions and parishes in London and other populous places, they have not thought it expedient in this Order to prohibit outdoor relief to any class of paupers.'

Accordingly it is required (1) that whenever the Guardians allow relief to any able-bodied male person out of the workhouse, one half at least of the relief so allowed shall be given in articles of food or fuel, or in other articles of absolute necessity.

(2) In resident cases, to prevent relief being squandered, or more being given than will provide against actual necessities, outdoor relief granted to an indigent poor person for more than one week must be given or administered weekly or oftener.

The Outdoor Test Regulation Order.

The Outdoor Relief Regulation Order:

Resident cases.

---

[1] What the able-bodied person receives is, it should be noted, not wages but relief. 'The object is "to provide a test of destitution," not primarily to get the largest return for the labour done. It is doubtless desirable that the paupers for the independent employment of whom either capital or inclination is wanting, should in return for their maintenance out of the rate be made to work, with as little loss to the union as possible, at some work in which they will not directly interfere with the independent labourer.'—Instructional letter re Outdoor Labour Test Order.

(3) 'The Guardians or their officers' are absolutely prohibited from using the poor-rates, directly or indirectly, to 'establish any applicant for relief in trade or business'; to 'redeem from pawn for any applicant any tools, implements, or other articles'; to purchase or give him any tools, implements, or other articles, except clothing or bedding when urgently needed, or 'food or fuel, or articles of absolute necessity'; to pay for the conveyance of any poor person, unless it be for the removal of a pauper to a workhouse, district school, &c.; to pay rent wholly or in part.

There are in regard to resident cases no restrictions, except in the case of able-bodied men.

The rules in regard to the relief of non-resident cases are the same as in the Prohibitory Order. (*See* p. xxxiii.) *The Outdoor Relief Regulation Order: Non-resident cases.*

The place of the Outdoor Relief Test Regulation Order is taken by clauses of a similar character:—

Thus, (1) 'No relief shall be given to any able-bodied male person while he is employed for wages or other hire or remuneration by any person.' *Out-Relief to the Able-bodied.*

(2) 'Every able-bodied male person, if relieved out of the workhouse, shall be set to work by the Guardians, and he kept employed under their direction and superintendence so long as he continues to receive relief.'

In cases of sudden and urgent necessity, sickness, &c., these requirements may, it is added, be dispensed with.

A comparison of the two Orders will show the indulgences which the Regulation Order permits in the Metropolis and other large towns. Thus, in these towns able-bodied women may receive outdoor relief; under the Prohibitory Order, except in cases of widowhood, they cannot. Again, under the Regulation Order, deserted wives may, if the Guardians so decide, receive outdoor relief; and further, several exceptions which, when the general rule is prohibitory, have an appearance of fairness and consideration, are of no importance one way or the other when the prohibition is withdrawn. Thus, where all may receive outdoor relief, there is no occasion for making an exception in the case of the wife of a soldier or sailor. So while sickness or urgency form a reasonable exception to the prohibitory rule, under the Regulation Order no such exceptions are required. That out-relief may be given in such cases goes without saying. *The Orders compared.*

From this statement in regard to outdoor relief, it follows that (as Mr. Goschen in his circular of 1869 pointed out) establishment in trade, taking goods out of pawn, purchasing tools, paying fares or rent, are, so far as the Poor Law is concerned, works of charity; but charity finds, for reasons which may have led to the Poor Law prohibitions, that these things (*e.g.* the payment of rent) can only be done by it with very great precaution. *Mr. Goschen's circular on Co-operation of Guardians with Charity.*

It is evident that very large discretion is given to the Guardians in the Metropolis in distinguishing between cases in which they grant indoor and those in which they grant outdoor relief, and that, by co-operation with the charitable, all cases, with which charity is better fitted to deal, may be taken up by it, while the Guardians relieve the remainder. It will be noted also that while there are many rules and restrictions respecting the able-bodied, there are none respecting the disabled—'the lame, impotent, old, blind, and such other among them being poor and not able to work,' though the limitation of the Act of Queen Elizabeth holds good, and in these cases only 'necessary relief' can be given. In regard to these the discretion of the Guardians is unfettered. Sometimes the Guardians give relief according to a scale, *e.g.* to a widow with so many children, so much in money and so many loaves. These scales, it may be well to mention, have no legal validity; they are adopted by the Guardians merely for their own convenience, to save the trouble of separate settlements of detail in each separate case. Their utility is very questionable.

XVa.—Pros and Cons as to Outdoor Relief.

Arguments for and against outdoor relief.

The question of the desirability of reducing out-relief is much debated. Some of the arguments in favour of doing so are, that it lacks the restrictive character of wholesome State relief; that it is looked upon as the recompense in old age of the pauper's payment of rates during life, and hence it weakens the inducements to thrift; that it is impossible to administer it on any large scale without encouraging deception, for the means of making an exhaustive investigation in a very large number of applications must necessarily be insufficient, and insufficient inquiry is a direct temptation to mis-statement and the concealment of material facts; that discrimination on moral or general grounds is hardly possible, and, even if it were, it would not be justifiable, as destitution is the sole test in Poor Law relief; that outdoor relief becomes a kind of inadequate and unsatisfactory supplementation of wages—tending to keep wages down; that it is no safeguard against starvation, for it is seldom sufficient to maintain the recipient, and for this reason, and on account of the difficulty of supervising constantly those who receive it, it is likely to cause rather than to prevent starvation; that it tempts the poor to neglect their relatives, since they will not come forward to help them if outdoor relief is given, but will do so if the 'house' is offered. Its advocates plead that the cost of a work-house system (quite apart from infirmaries for the sick and helpless) is excessive; that, whether or not it be expensive in the aggregate, it is so certainly case for case; that in this sense, at least, it is cheaper than indoor relief; that indoor relief is too punitive in its nature; that, since no reliance can be placed in charity—nor, indeed, should be, inasmuch as a State system should be self-sufficient—there is no satisfactory alternative to outdoor relief; that it is hard in most cases, directly or indirectly, to oblige the labouring poor to support their relations, since their wages can seldom be enough to meet their legitimate wants; that to diminish outdoor relief is a harsh measure, and will lead to a reaction in favour of a lavish administration, or even a general attack on the whole Poor Law system. On the whole, judging from the results of the system of restricting out-relief at St. George-in-the-East, Whitechapel, Stepney, Manchester, Birmingham, Bradfield, and elsewhere, the arguments against it appear to be conclusive.[1] There have, no doubt, been other causes at work besides good administration to produce the large reduction in pauperism that has taken place during the last 25 years, for prices have been low and wages have risen. Yet beyond question also in that period, with the constant discussion of methods of administration, administration itself has improved. The general decrease of pauperism has been very striking. It affects all classes of paupers alike, children, the able-bodied, and the aged. The population has increased since 1871 27·6 per cent.; nevertheless there is an actual numerical decrease in the number of child-paupers of 37 per cent.; and of 38 per cent. in the case of the able-bodied; and 18 per cent. in the case of the not able-bodied or infirm and aged.

In the Metropolis out-relief is discouraged by the arrangement by which the cost of it is thrown on the union, while the cost of indoor relief is borne by the Metropolitan Common Fund (*see* p. cxliii.).

By circular letters and in other ways the Local Government Board have tried to guide opinion in regard to the administration of outdoor relief; and different methods for its reduction or regulation have been adopted by different Boards of Guardians. One or two of these it may be well to mention.

First, there are the limitations in the administration of the Outdoor Relief Prohibitory and Regulation Orders, which have been officially approved by the Local Government Board as tending to a 'rigid and discriminating system of outdoor relief.'

1. As a general principle it is urged that instead of making the orders more stringent, ' it is competent for the Guardians to pass resolutions laying down the rules by which they will be guided in dealing with particular classes of cases.'

2. A circular issued in 1871 makes the following suggestions :— The circular of 1871.

(1.) That outdoor relief should not be granted to single able-bodied men, or to single able-bodied women, either with or without illegitimate children.

(2.) That outdoor relief should not, except in special cases, be granted to any woman deserted by her husband during the first twelve months after the desertion, or to any able-bodied widow with one child only.

(3.) That in the case of any able-bodied widow with more than one child it may be desirable to take one or more of the children into the workhouse in preference to giving outdoor relief.

---

[1] *See* various papers on ' Outdoor Relief,' published by the Charity Organisation Society.

(4.) That in unions where the Prohibitory Order is in force, the workhouse test should be strictly applied.

(5.) That outdoor relief should be granted for a fixed period only, which should not, in any case, exceed three months.

(6.) That all orders to able-bodied men for relief in the labour-yard should only be given from week to week.

(7.) That outdoor relief should not be granted in any case unless the relieving officer has, since the application, visited the home of the applicant, and has recorded the date of such visit in the relief application and report book. Cases in which the relieving officer has not had time to visit, should be relieved by him in kind only, or by an order for the workhouse.

(8.) That the relieving officer should be required to make at least fortnightly visits to the homes of all persons receiving relief on account of temporary sickness, and of able-bodied men receiving relief in the labour-yard, and to visit the old and infirm cases at least once a quarter; and the relieving officer should be required to keep a diary with the dates and results of his visits.

(9.) That the provisions with respect to the compulsory maintenance of paupers by relations legally liable to contribute to their support should be more generally acted upon.

(10.) That as the recommendation of medical officers for meat and stimulants are regarded as equivalent to orders for additional relief, they should in all cases be accompanied by a report from the medical officer in a prescribed form, setting forth the particulars of each case ascertained by personal inquiry.

(11.) That in the most populous unions it may be expedient to appoint one or more officers to be termed ' inspectors of out-relief,' whose duty it would be to act as a check upon the relieving officers, and ascertain also the circumstances connected with the recipients of relief. Such appointments have already been tried in Liverpool,[1] and found to answer very successfully.

3. Stress is also laid on three other most important points. The district of the relieving officer must not be so large as to prevent the thorough investigation of each individual case. The application and report book must be properly and completely filled up, so that the whole evidence is in writing and comes before the Guardians in a clear and sufficient manner. The relieving officers must be competent and painstaking, and must visit frequently. The following paragraphs state these points very clearly :—

' It is of essential importance to any sound system of outdoor relief that the relief districts should not be too large, or the number of relieving officers too small. If a relieving officer's district be too large, it will be impossible for him, however zealous and vigilant he may be, to investigate with sufficient care the case of each applicant for relief, or pauper in receipt of relief; and nothing can be more objectionable than that an officer should be compelled to perform his duty in a hurried and incomplete manner.[2]

'One cause of a lax administration[3] of outdoor relief, is the imperfect manner in which applications for relief are often presented by the relieving officers to the Guardians. This remark is intended to point amongst other things to the frequent omission to enter in the proper column of the application and report book the names of relations of applicants for relief who are legally liable for their support.

---

[1] [Now also at West Derby, Birmingham, Manchester, and elsewhere (1894).]
[2] Circular of 1871. Local Government Board Report, 1877-8.
[3] Memorandum of 1878.

'To ensure relief being strictly limited to the class for whom it is intended [those in actual destitution], it is only requisite that those who are entrusted with the administration of the law should, by diligent and minute inquiry, ascertain the exact condition and circumstances of each applicant, and to enable the Guardians to do this effectually, it is essential that they should have the aid of competent and painstaking relieving officers, whose districts should not be so extensive as to preclude them from visiting each recipient of relief at his own home, and at frequent intervals, in conformity with the regulations of the Board.'

4. Some other points are these [1] :—

(1.) Non-resident relief might, in the opinion of the Board, be almost entirely discontinued.

(2.) While disapproving a suggestion that the Prohibitory Order should be altered so as to make it illegal to grant relief in sudden and urgent cases for more than a month at a time, the Board state 'it will still be competent for the Guardians to limit the relief in those cases, where such a limitation may be properly imposed, and that without interference on the part of the Board.'

(3.) Another suggested alteration of the Prohibitory Order the Board declares impracticable, viz., that the exception allowing relief to widows within six months of their widowhood should be omitted. But they state: 'It may be that the period of six months now allowed is too long, but the President, as at present advised, is not prepared to shorten it, preferring that the Guardians should exercise their discretion in dealing with each case according to its merits.'

5. As an example of rules to be adopted by Guardians, the Local Government Board have more than once referred with approval to those adopted by the Manchester Board. They are as follows :— *Manchester outdoor relief rules.*

1. Outdoor relief shall not be granted or allowed by the Relief Committees (except in cases of sickness) to applicants of any of the following classes :—

(*a*) Single able-bodied men ;

(*b*) Single able-bodied women ;

(*c*) Able-bodied widows without children, or having only one child to support ;

(*d*) Married women (with or without families) whose husbands having been convicted of crime, are undergoing a term of imprisonment ;

(*e*) Married women (with or without families) deserted by their husbands ;

(*f*) Married women (with or without families) left destitute through their husbands having joined the militia, and being called up for training ;

(*g*) Persons residing with relatives, where the united income of the family is sufficient for the support of all its members, whether such relatives are liable by law to support the applicant or not.

2. Outdoor relief shall not be granted in any case for a longer period than 13 weeks at a time.

3. Outdoor relief shall not be granted to any able-bodied person for a longer period than six weeks at a time.

4. Outdoor relief shall not be granted on account of the sickness of the applicant, or any of his family, for a longer period than two weeks at a time, unless such sickness shall be certified in writing by the district medical officer as being likely to be of long duration, or to be of a permanent character.

5. When relief is allowed to a parent through the admission of a child or children into the Swinton Schools or the workhouse, such relief shall not be granted for a longer period than six months at a time; and if at the expiration of such period a continuance of the relief is required, the relieving officer shall visit and inquire into the circumstances of the parent, and bring the case up for reconsideration by the Relief Committee, in the same manner as if it were a case for outdoor relief.

[1] Memorandum of 1878.

The Paddington Rules. Other rules may also be mentioned. Those adopted by the Paddington Guardians are somewhat different, but they are of interest inasmuch as they turn upon the principle that (excepting in cases of emergency) outdoor relief should be given only in those cases in which charity would ordinarily and rightly step in. Accordingly, where these rules are adopted, if the charitable organisations of the union are ready to do their duty, outdoor relief must necessarily disappear and charity take on the work that elsewhere is often inadvertently undertaken by the Poor Law.

These rules are :— Outdoor relief may be granted only to such aged and infirm persons as (1) are deserving at the time of application, (2) have shown signs of thrift, (3) have no relations legally or morally bound to, and able to, support them, (4) are unable to obtain sufficient assistance from charitable sources, (5) are desirous of living out of the workhouse and can be properly taken care of.

Whitechapel Procedure. 6. In Whitechapel and St. George-in-the East, where outdoor relief has been reduced to a minimum, no general rules have been adopted, but rather a new practice has been introduced and adhered to for the last twenty years. This practice was thus described by Mr. Vallance in his evidence before the Select Committee of the House of Lords on Poor Relief :—

'Up to 1870 the system may be said to have been that of meeting apparent existing circumstances of need by small doles of outdoor relief; the indoor establishments—at that time consisting of a mixed workhouse for the adult sick and healthy poor, and a separate school at Forest Gate—being reserved for the destitute poor who voluntarily sought refuge in them. Able-bodied men who applied for relief on account of want of employment were set to work under the Outdoor Relief Regulation Order, and in return for such work were afforded outdoor relief in money and kind. Under this system the administration was periodically subjected to great pressure, so much so that the aid of the police had not unfrequently to be invoked to restrain disorder and afford necessary protection to officers and property. Police protection was even at times required for the Guardians during their administration of relief. The experience of the winter of 1869-70, however, was such as to lead the Guardians to review their position, and earnestly to aim at reforming a system which was felt to be fostering pauperism and encouraging idleness, improvidence, and imposture, whilst the "relief" in no true sense helped the poor. It was seen that voluntary charity largely consisted of indiscriminate almsgiving; that it accepted no definite obligation as distinct from the function of Poor Law relief; that the Poor Law was relied upon to supplement private benevolence; that the almsgivers too frequently were the advocates of the poor in their demands upon the public rates; and that both Poor Law and charity were engaged in the relief of distress much of which a thoughtless benevolence and a lax relief administration had created. This condition of things the Guardians resolved to amend. Looking forward to the ultimate possibility of laying down a broad distinction between "legal relief" and "charitable aid," and of interpreting the former as relief in the workhouse, or other institution, for the actually destitute, and the latter as personal sympathy and helpful charity, they began by gradually restricting outdoor relief in "out-of-work" cases, until they were able to suspend the Outdoor Relief Regulation Order entirely, and to apply strictly the principle of the Prohibitory Order. Thus, the labour-yard was in the course of the year (1870) closed, and it has not since been re-opened. In this process of restriction it was found that about one in ten of those who were offered indoor, in place of outdoor, relief entered the workhouse, and these, in turn, gradually withdrew themselves, so that eventually the indoor pauperism resumed its normal condition.'. . . ' Thus, in point of fact, we have been acting very much as if the Prohibitory Order applied to the Whitechapel Union.

. . . ' At present, by reason of the perfect understanding which exists between the Guardians and the Charity Organisation Society, and indeed workers for the poor generally, the Guardians are enabled to say to the sick man, if he is not in a benefit club, that he will be received into the infirmary. The infirmary now is a separate building, under medical administration equal, it may be said, to a general hospital. By admitting the man to the infirmary we take security for his early recovery, as well as for his early entrance into the labour market again. With regard to his family, as a rule where they have been struggling, and are really deserving, there is no difficulty whatever in finding charity available at once ; but otherwise we admit part of the family with him. We have never found a difficulty. The relieving officers have always been instructed to be on the alert lest charity should fail in its duty of looking after the family of a man in the infirmary ; but we have not found a case in which it has been necessary to interpose with relief in kind.'

In answer to the question—

' But must it not have to considerable extent the effect of discouraging thrift, inasmuch as the man can fairly look forward to his family being provided for in such cases, and therefore does not feel the necessity of making provision himself ? '

Mr. Vallance said :—

' I do not think that it can be regarded as a certainty of provision. The Charity Organisation Society, for instance. in the case of a man admitted to the infirmary or the workhouse, would make their usual inquiry, and it is those who have homes worth preserving, those who have given some evidence of having exercised thrift, that are assisted. In other cases the Charity Organisation Society would probably refuse help, so that there could be no certainty ; and where it was refused, then a portion of the family would be offered admission with the head of the family, the mother and the youngest child probably being left out, so that she might achieve independence if she could, and tide over the period of her husband's illness. So that it is not a uniform grant by the [Charity Organisation Society, or what I may term a system of Poor Law administration outside the Poor Law with the same certainty.'

As to widows, he said :—

' A widow with dependent children is first referred to the Charity Organisation Society, the relieving officer being authorised to meet any circumstances of urgent necessity by relief in kind. In some cases the Society may succeed in introducing the widow to service, or employment, or may, by the purchase of a mangle or sewing machine, afford her the means of achieving independence, or— succeeding in part only—the Society may refer the case back to the Guardians with a request that one or more children may be admitted into the district school. It should also be stated that 36 poor widows are employed in the infirmary as washers and scrubbers at w ekly wages. . . . The relief which the Guardians would not hesitate to afford temporarily to widows of respectable character is rendered unnecessary by the intervention of organised charity.'

And, answering the question whether this ' the whole of the support of widows of respectable character in your union is thrown on charity ? ' he replied :—

' Not the " support " so much as seeing to it that the poor woman is brought within reach of the friendship, the sympathy, the personal help which will enable her to achieve independence.' '

A quotation from a recent Annual Report of the London Charity

<hr>

' Evidence : Select Committee of the House of Lords. Poor Law Relief. 1888.

Organisation Society throws further light on the advantages of a policy of closely restricted outdoor relief:—

What should take the place of outdoor relief.

'One obstacle in the way of reform is the common argument that a large amount of charitable relief must already be forthcoming and available for the assistance of cases in receipt of outdoor relief, if the latter is to be withdrawn. At first sight this seems plausible, but the substitute for outdoor relief is not, unless in exceptional instances, charitable relief, but providence, thrift, and the enforcement of family responsibilities. The mass of the people have within their reach the means of relieving themselves and their dependents in a thousand and one small ways, just as they have the means of supplying themselves with food. The distribution of food is self-acting, and presses to meet the demands of the multitude. It organises itself. So to a very large extent would it be with the ordinary relief of the people if they were not arbitrarily interfered with by the State and by philanthropists. What others press to do for them they may naturally think it foolish to do for themselves; and petty charities, doles, and allowances, and petty outdoor relief, are but means of diverting them from duties which they, like others, will only perform under the natural constraints of life. Relief is not for ordinary but exceptional cases; not for the mere maintenance of its recipients, but for the removal and prevention of their distress.

'On this point the following figures, taken from Mr. Vallance's evidence, throw light.

Whitechapel and outdoor relief.

In 1869 the indoor paupers at Whitechapel numbered 1,232; in 1888, 1,264. In 1869 the outdoor numbered 4,135; in 1888, 1,312. The totals are thus (1869) 5,367; (1888) 2,576. The cost of relief in money and kind for the year was, in 1869, £7,458; in 1888, £117.

'From this it appears that some £7,300 formerly spent annually for outdoor relief has been set free. It is available (without an increase of the rates) for more salutary relief of other kinds, such as an improved infirmary, or a careful and educational supervision of the inmates of the workhouse. Or it is left in the ratepayers' pockets, and the community has the advantage of so much more expended on industry and commerce. On the other hand, those who received it before no longer ask for it. They are maintaining themselves, or are maintained by their friends and relations, to the extent of the £7,300 a year. To that amount, either the relief was not wanted, or by the natural distribution of private charities it has been silently and unostentatiously provided by the people at large. Exceptional cases (including pension cases) in which charitable relief is required are referred to the Whitechapel Charity Organisation Committee, and the payment of some portion of the £7,300 has thus been undertaken by charity. If out relief were reduced throughout the metropolis as it has been in Whitechapel, St. George-in-the-East, and Stepney, the outdoor paupers would number about 22,800 instead of 49,118, and the annual saving in outdoor relief would amount to about £100,000; and for the most part private charity, which happily lies beyond the ken of any institution, would be stimulated to make that sum good, so far as it was actually required at all, and could not be met by the honest exertion of the would-be recipients.'[1]

XV*b*.—THE ORGANISATION OF THE WORKHOUSE.

The Workhouse: its administration and arrangements.

What then is the organisation of the workhouse[2]? A large building now often built in the suburbs, used not so much for work as for residence. It is under the charge of a master and matron. Admission to it is given on an order from the Guardians, or on a provisional order from the Relieving

[1] Annual Report of the Charity Organisation Society, 1887-8.

[2] Formerly, the workhouse included separate wards or blocks for the sick asylum or infirmary, the school, and for casuals. Now, in London, and many other large towns, the infirmary is, with few exceptions, a separate building; the schools are separate; and in many instances the casual wards are separate.

Officer, or (now very seldom) from an Overseer, or from the Master 'in any case of sudden or urgent necessity.' All such cases are admitted irrespective of the settlement of the pauper—that is, irrespective of the question whether the Union in which he is relieved ought to bear the cost of his relief as one of their 'settled' population (*see* p. xlix.). There is a receiving ward, in which the pauper is examined by a medical officer, thoroughly cleansed, and clothed in the workhouse dress; his own dress is set aside and purified. He is searched also, and if he has money upon him it may be used for his maintenance.[1] If he is suffering from infectious or contagious disease he is placed in a special ward. In the workhouse there is a classification of paupers in separate wards :—Males —(1), the aged and infirm ; (2), the able-bodied from 15 years old upward ; (3), boys from 7 to 15 ; (4, 5, and 6), Females in three similar divisions ; and (7), one class of children under 7. Further classification is recommended to prevent the moral contamination of inmates. Mothers of children under 7 have access to them at all reasonable times. All have to attend meals, except the sick, children, persons of unsound mind, 'casual' poor, wayfarers, women suckling their children, and the aged and infirm. There is a fixed dietary ; and only the dietary food is allowed. The whole institution is managed on a system of rigorous routine.

It may be useful to add a few miscellaneous details. Able-bodied inmates may be employed as superintendents, and still are used to some extent as nurses, and the Master has, according to the words of the Order, to employ the able-bodied, train the youths, occupy the partially incapable, and allow no idleness. Separate accommodation may be provided for aged and infirm couples. (1) In the case of 'any two persons being husband and wife,' and 'either of them infirm, sick, or disabled by an injury, or above the age of 60 years,' the Guardians may, in their discretion, permit them to live together in the workhouse.[2] (2) But if both husband and wife are over the age of 60, they will not be compelled to live separate in the workhouse.[3] Any person may visit any pauper in the workhouse by permission of the Master, subject to 'conditions prescribed by the Guardians.' *(margin: Employment of Inmates. Separate Accommodation for Aged and Infirm Couples. Visits to Paupers in the Workhouse.)*

To keep discipline, the Master can punish offences according as the delinquent pauper is 'disorderly,' or 'refractory '; terms which are defined with great precision, so as to include in the former 13, and the latter eight definite offences. The former, the first of which is

---

[1] If any person who applies for relief at a workhouse or to a relieving officer, has at the time in his possession, or under his control, money or other property, he has to make 'correct and complete disclosure,' or he is liable to be punished as 'idle and disorderly' (*see* p. lxvi.), 11 & 12 Vict., c. 110, s. 10. And 'any person' who obtains relief 'by wilfully giving a false name, or making a false statement,' is so liable. 39 & 40 Vict., c. 61, s. 44.

[2] 39 & 40 Vict., c. 61 (1876), s. 10.

[3] 10 & 11 Vict., c. 109, s. 23. *See* Lumley: 'Divided Parishes and Poor Law Amendment Act.'

making 'any noise when silence is ordered,' are punishable by the
Master at his own discretion—by substituting a less satisfactory
diet for any time less than 48 hours. The latter are only punishable,
except in aggravated cases, by the direction of the Guardians, by
reducing or changing the diet, and by confinement for any term less
than 24 hours. The corporal punishment of adults is not allowed.

Leaving the Workhouse. If a pauper wishes to leave the workhouse, he must be allowed
to do so, provided that he gives a reasonable notice. If he has a
family, he has to take it with him. A pauper who has stayed for a
month in a workhouse is, after giving notice, detained 24 hours; if
within the month he has left the workhouse, or, as the phrase is,
'discharged himself' once or oftener, he is detained 48 hours; if
twice in two months, 72 hours.[1]

But these paragraphs concerning the workhouse would give an
altogether misleading impression if it were not added that the
infirmary or sick asylum, which is usually, in London, a large
hospital, built according to well-approved methods of construction
and provided with a nursing staff, is included under that name.
Of late years the institutions that bear the common name 'workhouse' have tended to become more and more the refuge of the
sick, the feeble, and the aged. For the aged there is a separate
dietary, and they have many minor comforts; while for the sick
in the Metropolis all reasonable requirements are usually met.

XV.—Poor Law Relief by way of Loan; and Recovery of Relief.

Recovery of Poor Law relief as a loan. Two important powers of the Guardians should be noted here:

(1) Relief given in accordance with the outdoor relief regulation
(December 14, 1852) may be given by way of loan to or on account
of any person over 21, or to his wife, or to any of his family under
the age of 16. The master or employer of the recipient can, in all
cases in which relief has been given as a loan, be required by a
justice, on application from the Guardians, to show cause why
wages due, or from time to time due to the recipient should not be
paid over in whole or in part to the Guardians; and the justice
can, if he think fit, taking into consideration the circumstances of
such poor person and his family, require the employer from such
wages to pay the debt to the Guardians direct by instalments or in
a lump sum as may be arranged.[2]

By these provisions the Guardians, if they can bestow sufficient
time on the individual case, may deal effectively with a large class

---

[1] It may be noted that, with the approval of the Local Government Board,
the workhouses in the Metropolis may be appropriated to different classes of cases
to be received from any of the metropolitan unions. (30 Vict., c. 6, s. 80, and
32 & 33 Vict., c. 63, s. 17.)

[2] Poor Law Amendment Act, 1834 (4 & 5 Will. IV., c. 76), s. 59.

of ineligible cases, in which the parent is to blame for his family's distress, or in which, in fairness to the community, the applicant should be required to pay for what he has received.

In regard to Medical Relief, it is stated that 'as the exact cost of it in any individual case cannot in general be severed from the total cost of medical relief in the Union, it does not seem to be such relief as can be given by way of loan. But in some Unions it is nevertheless so given.'[1]

(2) Guardians can recover[2] as a debt the cost of the relief or of part of the relief they have given in the previous twelve months, if a pauper has in his possession any money or valuable security. In the event of the pauper's death, they may be reimbursed for twelve months' expenditure and the cost of burial.

Recovery of Poor Law relief as a debt.

XVI.—SETTLEMENT AND REMOVAL.[3]

The words 'settlement' and 'removal' frequently occur in connection with Poor Law cases. They require some explanation. Here, too, it is convenient to give in the briefest terms some particulars with regard to the words 'parish' and 'union,' in reference to Poor Law relief.

By the Poor Law Act of Queen Elizabeth,[4] the relief and chargeability of the poor were limited to the area of the parish. In the reign of Charles II. a law was passed by which parishes, often of an unwieldy size, might be subdivided. This law was unfairly applied, in order to create what were called 'close' parishes, sections of parishes in which there were few paupers, and hence low rates, while hard by were parishes with many paupers and high

'Parish,' and 'Union.'

---

[1] Glen, p. 435 (ed. 1883).

[2] Poor Law Union Charges Act Amendment, 1849 (12 & 13 Vict., c. 103), s. 16.

[3] Some grave difficulties have to be met or allowed for in any attempt to put down shortly the leading features of the legal provisions regarding intricate subjects such as settlement and removal, and many others touched upon in this 'Introduction.' Decisions on cases are continually modifying the statute law. Sometimes, every word in the section of an Act is limited by conditions to be found elsewhere. There is thus, practically, no alternative between a lengthy and somewhat technical memorandum and a brief statement, which, omitting many details and reservations, cannot but be more or less misleading. Notwithstanding these objections, it has been thought well to adopt the latter course, rather than to omit all reference to these questions, or to deal with them so generally, that the information given would hardly be found even suggestive. The almoner is likely to pass by many important provisions altogether, unless they are brought to his notice, in the first instance, in some compendious form. But if once the suggestion is made to him, and his work shows him its practical bearing, he can, by reference to the proper authorities or to books, ascertain any further particulars that may be necessary, or what the requirements of the law more exactly are. It has been desired to make this 'Introduction' suggestive, and so far as the limits of space allow, detailed and accurate. To make it exhaustive would be impossible, and it must thus also be, in a measure, incorrect. A list of Books of Reference will be found on pp. cxcv.–cxcviii., and in the notes numerous references are given.

[4] 43 Eliz., c. 2.

rates. The Poor Law Commissioners (1834) introduced the system of unions, by which, while each parish supported its own poor, the workhouse was maintained by the parishes in union, each giving its quota towards the cost.

It was subsequently enacted, in 1848 and the years following,[1] that persons who acquired the status of irremovability, should be relieved from the 'common fund of the Union,' and with some other classes of paupers, such as destitute wayfarers, &c., they became 'union paupers.' And the basis upon which the common fund was assessed was altered. It had been based on the average expense incurred by each parish in the relief of its own poor, during the three years previous. It was now, and has since been based, on the annual value of the rateable property of each parish. In 1865 another great change was made. The relief of all paupers was thrown on the common fund of the union.[2] Concurrently with these changes, changes were made in regard to the position of the parish in questions of removability. It had been necessary that, to obtain irremovability by residence, the poor person should not reside outside the parish. Afterwards residence in any one or more parishes, in a single union, was computed to make up the period of residence that conferred irremovability.[3] Removability, therefore, depends on residence in a union. In the enactments with regard to settlement, the words defining the local area are 'parish,' 'parish or place,' 'parish or township'; and no change has been made in the law, similar to that with regard to removability, by which the union is substituted for the parish as the area of settlement. Yet the distinction between parish and union has in a great measure lapsed. Many parishes, of course, were not considered too small, or otherwise unsuitable for administrative purposes. They remained parishes, such as Kensington, Islington, and others. Many, again, were made parts of unions; e.g. St. Luke's, Clerkenwell, and Holborn, which have been formed into the Holborn Union.[4]

Settlement and Removal. Parliament, in the reign of Charles II., appears to have been apprehensive of the undue growth of large towns, and of the diseases incident to a crowded population; and it was desirous of checking vagrancy, and of regulating, and as a result, of checking also, the circulation of labour.[5] It therefore made a law enabling

[1] Irremovable Poor Act, 1861 (24 & 25 Vict., c. 55), s. 8.

[2] Union Chargeability Act, 1865 (28 & 29 Vict., c. 79), s. 2.

[3] The case of a deserted wife is an exception. She must continue to reside in the same parish as that in which she lived when deserted, to gain exemption from removal. See p. xlviii. (6).

[4] See the Poor Removal and Chargeability Acts, by W. G. Lumley. Knight & Co., Fleet Street, 1865. A short paper, 'Poor Removal within the Metropolis,' by Mr. Robert W. Monro, a guardian at Paddington, will be found of interest, in regard to the present state of this question in London.

[5] 14 Charles II., c. 12. See 'History of the English Poor Law,' by Sir George Nicholls, vol. I., p. 293.

justices, under certain conditions, to send back to their homes—to the place of their last settlement—persons who were likely to become chargeable to the parish. A procedure which had been previously introduced for dealing with vagrants only, was thus extended to the ordinary poor. By a later statute this power of the justices was limited to persons who became actually chargeable.[1] Since then many modifications have been made (see below) by which a right of irremovability is secured to persons who are residing in and become chargeable to a parish or union,[2] in which they have not a settlement. The result of the law of Charles II. has thus been that two series of questions have to be asked by the Guardians, in the case of every pauper: can we remove him, or must we pay for him here? and, if we can remove him, where is the place of his last settlement? Further, by successive enactments it has come about that, while residence, under certain conditions, confers irremovability, the same residence does not confer settlement. If, therefore, the Guardians have to pay for the relief of a pauper, because he is irremovable, they are no less interested in securing that, if he leaves their union, he should leave it without having contracted there a right of settlement; for in the event of his requiring relief, before he has acquired any new right of irremovability in the union to which he goes, he will be sent back, not to them, but to the place of his last settlement, the place to which, on his becoming chargeable, they would themselves have removed him if the law had allowed them to do so. The question of removal and settlement is, it is obvious, intricate, whether for purposes of administration or to the student. One set of conditions govern ' irremovability,' and another ' settlement.' A person who is settled in the union in which he becomes chargeable, is, of course, irremovable from it; but many that are irremovable from the union in which they become chargeable, are not settled in it.

Under what circumstances, then, is a person who becomes chargeable to a parish, not to be removed; when is he ' irremovable '? *Removal.*

(1) He cannot be removed, if he is legally settled where he is (see below).

(2) If he has resided in the union without interruption for one year next before the application for a warrant of removal, he cannot be removed.[3] *Irremovability by residence.*

(3) A child under 16, left an orphan, while residing with its surviving parent, cannot be removed, if the parent at the time of death was exempt from removal by reason of length of residence.[4] *Orphans under 16.*

[1] 35 Geo. III., c. 101. s. 1.
[2] 14 Charles II., c. 12. See ' History of the English Poor Law,' by Sir George Nicholls, vol. I p. 293.
[3] 28 & 29 Vict., c. 79, s. 8. See as to the definition and conditions of residence, Glen's Poor Law Statutes, vol. II. p. 815, 1873; see also W. G. Lumley's Poor Removal and Union Chargeability Acts.
[4] 24 & 25 Vict., c. 55, s. 2.

Children under 16.

(4) No child under 16, whether legitimate or illegitimate, residing in any parish with father or mother, stepfather or stepmother, or reputed father, can be removed, unless the parent can also be lawfully removed.[1]

A child cannot be removed from its parent if it be under the age of seven years, which is called the age of nurture; and if it become chargeable and have a different settlement from its parent, it must, nevertheless, be allowed to remain with the parent until it attain the age of seven years, or if the parent be removed, it must be removed also, to the same parish.[2]

Wife and children.

(5) If a wife becomes chargeable in the absence of her husband she may be removed to his last legal settlement, if he has one, or if not, then to the place of her maiden settlement.[3] Children and wife are only removable with the father and husband.

Deserted wife.

(6) If a deserted wife continues to reside for one year in the same parish in such a manner as would, if she were a widow (see next clause), render her exempt from removal, she is not liable to removal unless her husband returns to live with her.[4]

Widows.

(7) A widow residing in any parish with her husband at the time of his death, cannot be removed for twelve calendar months after, if she so long remains a widow.[5] Also 'non-resident relief' may (7 & 8 Vict., c. 101, s. 26) be given by the Guardians of the union of her settlement to a widow who continues on her husband's death to reside in the union where he died. The widow, in such a case, must have a legitimate child dependent on her for support, and no illegitimate child born after the commencement of widowhood.

(8) Persons who become chargeable for relief received owing to sickness or accident are not removable, unless they are likely, in the opinion of the justices, to become permanently disabled.[6] When they are cured they become chargeable to their own union.

It should be noted that persons exempted from removal do not by reason of such exemption acquire any settlement.[7] Also in computing the length of residence there must be excluded—among other exceptions—the time during which a person is in prison, or in an asylum, or hospital.[8]

The Guardians, if satisfied as to the facts of settlement, arrange for the removal or reception of paupers to or from other unions. But in cases of dispute a removal order is made by two justices on the complaint of the Guardians.

If a pauper, removed by a removal order, returns and becomes

---

[1] 9 & 10 Vict., c. 66, s. 3.   [2] Glen's Archbold, p. 571.
[3] Glen's Archbold, p. 565.   [4] 29 & 30 Vict., c. 113, s. 17.
[5] 9 & 10 Vict., c. 66, s. 2, and Glen's Archbold, p. 594.
[6] 9 & 10 Vict., c. 66, s. 4 ; 24 & 25 Vict., c. 5, s. 55.
[7] Ibid., s. 5 ; and 28 & 29 Vict., c. 79, s. 13.   [8] Ibid., s. 1.

chargeable within twelve months he is liable to be convicted and punished as 'idle and disorderly' (*see* p. lxvi.).[1]

If, then, a person may be removed, the next question is where may he be removed to ? Where is the place of his last settlement ? What constitutes settlement ?

Settlements are said to be of two kinds—original, when the person has acquired it himself; derivative, when he has acquired it indirectly, *e.g.* as a child by parentage, a wife by marriage. The only derivative settlements now recognised are as follows :[2]

(1) A wife acquires on marriage the settlement of her husband, if he have one. She cannot while married acquire any separate settlement of her own.

(2) A child under the age of 16 takes the settlement of its father or widowed mother, which it retains until it acquires another settlement.

(3) An illegitimate child retains the settlement of its mother until it acquires another settlement.

Of original settlements there are the following amongst others :

(4) Residence for three years 'in any parish in such manner and under such circumstances as would, in accordance with statutes in that behalf, render a person irremovable,' gives settlement,[3] until settlement in some other parish may be acquired.

(5) The occupation for one year of a tenement, being a separate and distinct dwelling-house of a not less annual value than £10, for which the occupant has been assessed, and has paid poor-rate for one year, gives settlement.[4]

(6) The owner of an estate in land, however small in value, by a residence of forty days in the parish in which it is situated, acquires a settlement.[5]

Questions of settlement are often of practical interest to the almoner. Thus, to the displeasure of the Guardians, a charitable institution may attract from other unions incurable or other inmates, who by residence become irremovable. This has often been a matter of complaint. Again, if assistance is wanted from the Guardians for an idiot or epileptic child, whose mother, a widow, has removed to another union in which she is not 'settled,' the Guardians may refuse to assist her child. She may return, they may say, to her proper union.[6] The decision as to whether the

Margin notes: Settlement. Wife. Children under 16. Illegitimate child. Settlement by residence. By occupation. By estate. Interest of charity in questions of settlement and removal.

---

[1] 28 & 29 Vict., 79, s. 7.
[2] Poor Law Amendment Act 1876 (39 & 40 Vict., c. 61), s. 35.
[3] 39 & 40 Vict., c. 61, s. 34. *See* Poor Law Amendment Act 1876, with notes, by E. Lumley, 1876.
[4] *See* Glen's Archbold, pp. 498 and 615. [5] Glen's Archbold, p. 499, etc.
[6] Residence in a charitable institution does not confer settlement, but such residence is no bar to contracting irremovability. In 1882 a 'Settlement of Removal Law Amendment Bill' was brought in by the Government. It was proposed to reduce settlement by residence from three years to one, and irremovability by residence from one year to three months.

child should be assisted, and the cost of relief, will then fall upon the Guardians of the union of her settlement.

XVII.—THE LEGAL RESPONSIBILITIES OF RELATIONS.

Any relief which removes a natural obligation is in its results of very doubtful benefit. The law according to its letter at least fully recognises this. Charity often forgets it. The issue is fairly raised in such a case as that mentioned on p. cv.

Why the obligations of relations should be enforced. Money given in such an instance is only spent in drink; and the removal of the child sets the parent free to indulge himself without fear of consequences. It may be urged that the child should be saved; and the plea is a strong one. But, unless the case be exceptional, the effect on the class will be bad : existing ties and responsibilities are none too numerous to keep men to their duty. What a man sees done for his neighbour, he thinks he is entitled to himself, and he yields to self-indulgence, well aware that there is charity in the background and in the last resort the Poor Law. There is abundant evidence in proof of this. Whenever it is possible, therefore, the relations should be required to do their part. The disgrace of leaving the fulfilment of their duty to strangers should be insisted on, and a definite scheme of help should be submitted to them, with a request for assistance of a definite kind or to a definite amount. No trouble should be spared to reassert the family bond.

The law deals with the question very precisely; a knowledge of it may enable the almoner to push relations to the alternative which they often dread, of letting those for whom they are legally or morally liable 'go on the rates,' or assisting them. The moral and pecuniary result of the enforcement of the law against relations, is shown in a return kindly furnished by the Clerk of the Barton Regis Union, near Bristol. In the year ended March 1870, £242. 15s. was received from relations and friends. During that and previous years only those paid who offered to do so. But in the nineteen years ended March 1889, £26,831 were received from relatives; £1,719 was received in 1880–81; £2,247 in 1889. 'These figures represent *the cash actually received*, but cases often occur,' the return states, ' where the relations, on notice being given them that proceedings are about to be commenced, maintain the pauper rather than submit to proceedings. The relief saved in such cases is considerable. The amount now collected in excess of 1870 pays the salaries of all the Clerks and Relieving Officers, which were previously a heavy charge upon the ratepayers.' Other Boards of Guardians act more or less persistently on the same plan. The St. Pancras Parish recover about £2,000 a year from relatives and friends of persons chargeable. In 1859 the Wandsworth Union collected from this source £1,667 : in 1885 the corresponding sum was £1,042.

(1) **Parents, Grandparents, and Children.**—With the exceptions mentioned below, all related within these degrees are, under the Act of Queen Elizabeth, 43, c. 2, s. 6[1], on an order by justices in petty sessions, liable for the maintenance of the others; but on two conditions: (*a*) That the relation to be maintained is 'a poor, blind, lame and impotent person or other person *unable to work.*' Inability to work is a *sine quâ non*. (*b*) That the relation that should maintain him is, in the opinion of the justices, ' of *sufficient ability*' to do so, at the time when they make their order. What the manner and rate of maintenance are to be the justices have to assess. If there be non-compliance with their order, the defendant forfeits 20*s*. a month so long as the non-compliance lasts.[2]

The Act 'extends only to natural relations, that is to say, to cases where there is relationship by blood between the parties, to lawful and not to reputed parents or children. And therefore under the statute a man cannot be compelled to contribute to the maintenance of his wife's mother, or his wife's child by a former husband, or her illegitimate child—after the wife's death, or after such child has attained the age of sixteen; or of his son's wife or widow; or of his own brother, a brother not being mentioned in the statute. But a grandfather is liable to contribute thus to the maintenance of his grandchild, even although the father be alive, if the latter be unable to support him; or indeed whether the father be unable or not; and, therefore, in such an order against a grandfather, it is not necessary to state that the father is dead or unable to support his children; but under 43 Eliz., c. 2, s. 6, a grandchild is not liable to maintain a grandfather.' [3]

'A grandmother under coverture is not liable to maintain her grandchild, notwithstanding that she has separate estate and is of "sufficient ability." The 21st section of the Married Women's

---

[1] The wording of the statute, Eliz., c. 2, is: 'The father and grandfather, and the mother and grandmother, and the children of every poor, old, blind, and impotent person, or other person not able to work, being of sufficient ability, shall, at their own charges, relieve and maintain every such poor person, in that manner, and according to that rate, as shall be assessed by the justices; upon pain that every one of them shall forfeit twenty shillings for every month which they shall fail therein.'

[2] In Stone's Justice's Manual there is the following suggestive note:—'The condition of the labouring class was such in A.D. 1601 that it cannot be considered labourers were included, or were intended to be included, as of "sufficient ability" in the Statute of Queen Elizabeth, which imposed a penalty of one pound a month (the equivalent of five pounds a month of our present money) in case of failure to perform the order. We doubt whether persons of that class, earning the ordinary weekly wages of thirteen shillings and fourteen shillings a week, are within these Statutes, which ought to be strictly interpreted. An application to quash such an order was made to the Queen's Bench in Hilary Term, 1876, but the proceedings failed, because the *certiorari* was not applied for within six months of the date of the order. The hearing of that order was not reported. [Parsley's case, 39 J P. 795].' The orders must be enforced as civil debts.

[3] Glen's Archbold, p. 221.

Property Act provides that a married woman shall be subject to all such liability for the maintenance of her children and grandchildren as the "husband is now by law subject to for the maintenance of *her* children and grandchildren." There can be no doubt that it was intended to make a woman who has married a second husband liable for the maintenance of her grandchildren. but as a husband is not bound to maintain a second wife's grandchildren. and she is only liable to the same extent, it would seem that she is still not bound to maintain her grandchildren.'[1]

'The marriage of the mother does not relieve her children by a former marriage from liability to maintain her, whilst she is living with her second husband.'[1]

An illegitimate child does not come within the Act, nor the father or the mother of an illegitimate child.

(2) Husbands, their Wives and Children.—Relief given by the Guardians to wife or to children, not being deaf, dumb, or blind, till they reach the age of 16, or on their account, is considered as given to the husband. A husband is liable to maintain his wife's children, legitimate or illegitimate, born before marriage,[2] until the age of 16, or the death of their mother, and he is chargeable with all relief granted to them. Any persons wilfully refusing or neglecting to maintain themselves or their families when able to do so wholly or in part, are liable to imprisonment and hard labour for a term not exceeding one month.[3] Desertion of wife and children, if they are left chargeable to the parish, is punishable by imprisonment and hard labour for a term not exceeding three months.[4] The property, if any, of the husband is available for the maintenance by the Guardians of his wife and children. Any parent who neglects to provide adequate food, clothing, medical aid, or lodging for his child being in his custody under the age of 14, whereby the health of the child has been, or is likely to be, seriously injured, is liable to be imprisoned for six months with or without hard labour.[5] In these cases 'the Guardians of the union or parish in which such child may be living shall institute the prosecution and pay the costs thereof out of their funds.' It does not appear to be necessary that the child should be chargeable, before the Guardians take action. So long as it may appear that a husband is beyond the seas, or in custody of the law, or confined as a lunatic or idiot, relief given to the wife, or to her children, is given to her as if she were a

Marginal notes:
Liability of husband.

Wife desertion.

Neglect of children.

Liability of husband and wife.

---

[1] Stone's Justice's Manual, edited by George B. Kennett, pp. 684, 685, ed. 1893

[2] 4 & 5 Will. IV., c. 76, ss. 56 & 57.

[3] 5 Geo. IV., c. 83, s. 3, and Glen's Poor Law Statutes, p. 431 ; cf. also Stone's Justice's Manual (1893), p. 957.

[4] 5 Geo. IV., c. 83, s. 4, and Glen's Poor Law Statutes, p. 433; Addenda.

[5] 31 & 32 Vict., c. 122, s. 37, and Glen's Poor Law Statutes, p. 1335. The Prevention of Cruelty to Children Act 1894, very largely increases the possibility of proceeding against persons who have the custody, charge, or care of children under 16, for neglect and other offences. *See* p. xcix.

widow, and she is considered responsible for the maintenance of her family; but the obligations and liabilities of the husband are in no way diminished by this.[1] A woman living separate from her husband is similarly responsible;[2] and if she have separate property, she 'shall be liable for the maintenance of her children and grandchildren, in like manner as her husband is liable, but he is not thereby relieved from his liability in that respect.' (*See* also as to grandmother under coverture, above.) When a married woman applies to the Guardians for relief without her husband, he may be summoned and required to pay towards the cost of the relief of his wife.[3] On the other hand, the wife is liable for the support of her husband, and, having separate property, for the support of her children. This does not, however, relieve the husband of his responsibilities in any way. Widows are liable for the relief given to their children, until the age of 16.[4]

(3) Illegitimate Children.—In the case of illegitimate children, an affiliation order may be made by justices in petty sessions charging the putative father to pay expenses incidental to the child's birth, or for its funeral, and any sum not exceeding 5s. a week to support and educate it till it reaches the age of 13 or 16. The Guardians can summon the putative father if, and so long as, the child is chargeable to the parish.[5] The mother of an illegitimate child is bound to maintain it until the child is 16, or acquires a settlement in its own right, or till it marries, if a female, or till the mother

Illegitimate children.

[1] 7 & 8 Vict., c. 101, s. 25.
[2] 39 & 40 Vict., c. 61, s. 18. *See* E. Lumley's Poor Law Amendment Act 1876, p. 12. This does not apply to cases of desertion. *Cf.* Married Women's Property Act 1882 (45 & 46 Vict., c. 75), s. 21.
[3] 31 & 32 Vict., c. 122, s. 33.   [4] 4 & 5 Will. IV., c. 76, s. 56.
[5] Two notes may be added : (1) as to the procedure adopted by Guardians ; (2) that to be adopted by any single woman.
(1) When a bastard child becomes chargeable to a union or parish, the Guardians may apply to any two justices, having jurisdiction in the union or parish, in petty sessions. This application may be made at any time when the child becomes chargeable and is under the age of 13. Thereupon the justices may summon the man alleged to be the father of the child to appear before any two justices having the like jurisdiction, to show cause why an order should not be made upon him to contribute towards the relief of the child, and upon his appearance, or on proof that the summons was duly served on him, or left at his last place of abode, six days at least (*i.e.* clear days) before the petty sessions, the justices in such petty sessions shall hear the evidence of the mother, and such other evidence as she or the Guardians may produce, and shall also hear any evidence tendered by or on behalf of the man alleged to be the father, and, if the evidence be corroborated in some material particular by other evidence to the satisfaction of the justices, they may adjudge the man to be the putative father, and make an order on him to pay what shall appear to them proper. (*f.* Stone's Justice's Manual, p. 168.
(2) 35 & 36 Vict., c. 65, s. 3. 'Any single woman (married woman living apart from her husband, or widow) may apply to any justice' acting for the place in which she is resident, 'for a summons, to be served on the man alleged to be the father of the child, in respect of which she applies ; also a woman not cohabiting with her husband, may, upon sufficient evidence of non-access, founded on other testimony than her own, make a similar application ; but

marries[1]; and 'any woman neglecting to maintain her bastard child, being able wholly or in part so to do, whereby such child becomes chargeable, is punishable as *an idle* and *disorderly* person ; and for a second offence, or for deserting her bastard child, whereby it becomes chargeable, as a rogue and vagabond ' (Poor Law Amendment Act 1844, 7 & 8 Vict., c. 101, s. 6.)[2]

(4) Deserted Children.—By the Poor Law Act 1889 (52 & 53 Vict., c. 56), the Guardians may by resolution assume control over a deserted child until the age of 16.

The main section of this Act is as follows :—

'Where a child is maintained by the Guardians of any Union, and was deserted by its parent, the Guardians may at any time resolve that such child shall be under the control of the Guardians until it reaches the age, if a boy, of sixteen, and, if a girl, of eighteen years, and thereupon until the child reaches that age all the powers and rights of such parent in respect of that child shall, subject as in this Act mentioned, vest in the Guardians: Provided that the Guardians may rescind such resolution if they think that it will be for the benefit of the child to be either permanently or temporarily under the control of such parent, or of any other relative, or any friend.'

A court of summary jurisdiction, if satisfied, on complaint of the parent, that the child has not been maintained by the Guardians, or deserted, or that it is for the benefit of the child to be permanently or temporarily under the control of the parent, may make an order determining the resolution of the Guardians.

'Maintained by the Guardians' is defined as 'wholly or partly maintained by them in a workhouse or in any district school, separate school, separate infirmary, sick asylum, hospital for infectious diseases, institution for the deaf, dumb, blind, or idiots, or any certified school under 25 and 26 Vict., c. 43, or boarded-out by the Guardians, whether within or without the limits of the Union.'

'Where a parent is imprisoned under a sentence of penal servitude or imprisonment in respect of an offence committed against a child.' the section of the Act applies as if the child had been deserted. The liability of parents to contribute towards the child's maintenance remains intact. A provision is added to safeguard the religious education of the child in accordance with its own creed.

(5.) Children deserted or abandoned, or brought up at the expense of some other person, school or institution, or Board of Guardians.—The power of the parent over a child is, under certain circumstances, still further limited by the Custody of Children Act 1891.

she cannot, in other cases, thus relieve her husband from the duty of maintaining her illegitimate child, whether born or begotten before their marriage.' . . . . Should the woman's application ' be delayed for more than a year after the birth, it will be too late, unless she be in a position to support it by a declaration upon oath that the alleged father has, during that twelvemonth, paid money towards the child's maintenance.' *See* The Justice's Note Book, by W. Knox Wigram, p. 99.

[1] 4 & 5 Will. IV., c. 76, s. 71. As to husband's responsibilities in regard to his wife's illegitimate children, *see* p. lii.

[2] *See* Stone, p. 960 (1893), notes.

This Act applies to children being brought up by another person than the parent—'person' including any school or institution—or by a Board of Guardians. It is not limited, therefore, to cases in which Boards of Guardians only are concerned, but it may be conveniently quoted here. Its main sections are as follows :—

'1. Where the parent of a child [*i.e.* any person at law liable to maintain such child or entitled to his custody] applies to the High Court or the Court of Session for a writ or order for the production of the child, and the Court is of opinion that the parent has abandoned or deserted the child, or that he has otherwise so conducted himself that the Court should refuse to enforce his right to the custody of the child, the Court may in its discretion decline to issue the writ or make the order.
(margin: Power of Court as to production of child.)

'2. If at the time of the application for a writ or order for the production of the child the child is being brought up by another person,' or is boarded-out by the Guardians of a Poor Law union, or by a parochial board in Scotland, the Court may, in its discretion, if it orders the child to be given up to the parent, further order that the parent shall pay to such person, or to the Guardians of such Poor Law union, or to such parochial board, the whole of the costs properly incurred in bringing up the child, or such portion thereof as shall seem to the Court to be just and reasonable, having regard to all the circumstances of the case.
(margin: Power to Court to repayment of costs of bringing up child.)

'3. Where a parent has—
'(a) abandoned or deserted his child; or
'(b) allowed his child to be brought up by another person at that person's expense, or by the Guardians of a Poor Law union, for such a length of time and under such circumstances as to satisfy the Court that the parent was unmindful of his parental duties;
the Court shall not make an order for the delivery of the child to the parent unless the parent has satisfied the Court that, having regard to the welfare of the child, he is a fit person to have the custody of the child.
(margin: Court in making order to have regard to conduct of parent.)

'4. Upon any application by the parent for the production or custody of a child, if the Court is of opinion that the parent ought not to have the custody of the child, and that the child is being brought up in a different religion to that in which the parent has a legal right to require that the child should be brought up, the Court shall have power to make such order as it may think fit to secure that the child be brought up in the religion in which the parent has a legal right to require that the child should be brought up. Nothing in this Act contained shall interfere with or affect the power of the Court to consult the wishes of the child in considering what order ought to be made, or diminish the right which any child now possesses to the exercise of its own free choice.'
(margin: Power to Court as to child's religious education.)

On this Act we have received the following useful comment, which we reprint :—

'The Custody of Children Act 1891 does not confer on a Board of Guardians any power to adopt a child; what it does is to diminish the right of a parent, in certain cases, to have his child given up to him, if he applies to the Court for the purpose. Thus if in the case of a parent of idle or vicious habits, or who is constantly in and out of the workhouse, the Guardians refused to give up his child to him and he applied to the Court to compel them to give it up, the Court might, in their discretion, refuse to do so, if they were of opinion (1) that he had abandoned, or deserted the child, or (2) that he had otherwise so conducted himself that they should refuse to enforce his right to the custody of the child. Moreover, if the parent had abandoned or deserted the child, or had allowed it to be brought up by another person at that person's expense, or by the Guardians for such a length of time and under such circumstances as to satisfy the Court that he was unmindful of his parental duties, the Court must not make an order for the delivering of the child to him unless he satisfies them that, having regard to the welfare of the

¹ 'Person' includes any school or institution.

child, he is a fit person to have the custody of it. It will be seen that the Act does not directly give powers to the Guardians, but it practically enables the Court to exercise a discretion as to whether the child shall be given up in the cases coming within its terms, if application is made to them to order this to be done. Moreover, if they make the order they have certain powers for directing the parent to repay the costs incurred in bringing up the child.'

XVIII.—DESERTED WOMEN.

Charity should not, as a rule, assist deserted women.

The legal obligations of husbands have been just referred to (*see* p. lii.). As soon as a deserted woman, or her child or children, become chargeable to the parish, the Guardians may proceed against the husband. Formerly (under 5 Geo. IV., c. 83, s. 4) proceedings had to be taken within six months; they may now be taken within two years after the commission of the offence.[1] (*See* also below, Section XXX., 'Married Women '—desertion.) As a rule the cases of deserted women may be considered ineligible for charitable help for the following reasons: the Guardians have this ready means of enforcing the husband's obligation; there is often collusion between the husband and wife; the offer of the ' house ' is a wholesome check in wife-desertion, for the husband is likely to dread for his wife and children the alternative between the workhouse and desertion, but not the alternative between desertion and charity or out-relief. Speaking at a meeting of the North-Western District Conference of Poor Law Guardians, Mr. Henley, then one of the general inspectors of the Local Government Board, said: ' Before 1871 there was a very general disposition on the part of Boards of Guardians, in the centre of England at any rate, to give out-relief to deserted women. A conference was held to consider the question, and after immense discussion the Conference came to the conclusion that deserted women should be relieved only in the workhouse. The consequence was that they rarely heard now of women deserted by their husbands. There used to be more women deserted by their husbands in Birmingham than in any other place in the kingdom. He did not say that desertion had decreased, but he did say that the cases of desertion which came before the Guardians had entirely disappeared. Because, what did the Guardians do? They spared neither time nor money to bring the men to justice, and the end of it was that these applications were put an end to altogether.'[2]

XIX.—FALLEN WOMEN.

A very large proportion of the mothers of illegitimate children have recourse to the Union Infirmary. In these, as in other cases, the first question is, not ' Is this person " deserving " ? ' but ' Can

[1] Poor Law Amendment Act 1876 (39 & 40 Vict., c. 61), s. 19, E. Lumley, p. 12.

[2] *See* Report of Fourteenth Annual Poor Law Conference for the North-Western District, October 1888. (Knight & Co., Fleet Street.) Principles of Decision, Charity Organisation Paper, No. 5, p. 4.

we in this instance effect an improvement or cure?' If the answer is in the affirmative, charity will be guided by the special character and tendencies of the individual, and help may be given to good purpose. The usefulness of a Workhouse Girls' Aid Committee such as those at Kensington and elsewhere for helping them was shown on p. xxiv. No doubt many may rightly be intercepted by charity and never 'go on the rates.' But as there must be a quality of sternness in the kindness that is to stamp out vice, and as the Poor Law has properly no preventive functions, it is right that as a rule the Poor Law should deal with these cases. It may thus afford temporary maintenance for the mother and permanent maintenance for the child while it requires both parents to support their offspring; and charity may step in to do what the Poor Law cannot do—to replace, in a position of respectability and self-dependence, the person who has, in a manner, been punished by the disgrace of the Poor-Law relief. Natural obligations may thus remain unimpaired. For such difficult work the most careful personal charity is requisite. If the charitable were to make the Infirmaries in the Metropolitan Unions centres for work of this kind, many lives made hopeless by pressure of circumstances and by association with vice would be saved, when a fresh start—downwards or upwards—must be made.

XX.—Inebriates.

It is generally allowed that intemperance is the cause of a large part of the crime and pauperism of this country. As a rule cases of intemperance, especially if the intemperance be of long standing, must be left to the Poor Law. The able-bodied man may reduce his family to misery, but so long as he is in receipt of wages neither he nor his children have any claim on the Poor Law. Habitual intemperance is not yet considered a penal offence, or, like lunacy, a malady so harmful to others that it must be subjected to State control, though in the Habitual Drunkards Act, and in the section, referred to below, of the Act for the Prevention of Cruelty to Children 1894, we find methods which may be extended into a system of State intervention, without requiring, as at present, the consent of the individual concerned, in cases in which intemperance leads to the neglect or injury of children, servants, or apprentices. If charity is given, the drunkard is only set free to indulge himself the more. At last, however, when drink has led to destitution, the case falls to the Poor Law. Much might be done by personal influence before the intemperance has become habitual, if religious and moral agencies were so organised as to take charge of individual cases for a period. This at present they are seldom able to do. 'Retreats,' managed under improved conditions and at less cost, would be very useful.

The Habitual Drunkards Act (1879), amended by a further Act in 1888, established a system of 'retreats.' Justices of the Peace in special or quarter sessions can give licenses to keep retreats for thirteen months at a time. The keepers are responsible for the management and have to reside in the retreats, to each of which a duly qualified medical man must be attached. For their supervision there is an Inspector of Retreats, who has to visit them twice a year and report. Any habitual drunkard may apply to the licensee or keeper of the retreat for admission, signing a statement that he will conform to regulations and remain in the retreat a certain time. Two persons have also to make a declaration that they are satisfied that the applicant is an habitual drunkard and understands the effect of the application. Then two Justices of the Peace have to attest the applicant's signature, on the same two conditions. The applicant cannot then leave the retreat till the time fixed for his detention has elapsed, unless he is discharged by order of a Justice. If in the retreat he neglects or wilfully refuses to conform to the rules, he may, on summary conviction, be fined 5l. or imprisoned 7 days; any person thinking himself aggrieved may appeal to quarter sessions. Very little has yet been done to take advantage of this legislation. There are at present only eight homes certificated under the Act, and the admissions in 1893 numbered only 129. The reports from the Licensees of Homes published in the last annual report of the Inspector show that the stay of the patients is often far too short to make it possible to effect a cure of the disease, while at some homes, as, for instance, that at Twickenham, 'fully 50 per cent. of the admissions are suffering from disease other than or in addition to the liquor habit.' The managers of the Rickmansworth home write:—

'To be effectual, legislative measures must be on a broader and more liberal basis; (1) To include power of committal by justices of criminal inebriates to special institutions for detention and curative treatment. (2) To apply more completely to *non-criminal* inebriates in so far as to maintain a voluntary section, which should be as purely voluntary and free from objectionable procedure as possible; and compulsory powers applicable to those cases who—although incapable of managing themselves or their affairs—are still unwilling to place themselves under protection and curative influence. (3) Provision for the poorer classes. (4) Safeguards should be provided amply sufficient for the protection of the liberty of the subject, and all interests bearing upon the individual, his relatives, and the public. Finally, all legislative provisions should be framed with the object of treating a morbid mental condition; this principle forms the basis of the whole question. Typical inebriety is a diseased condition closely allied to, if not an actual form of, insanity. The craving for liquor in an inebriate is an impulse as strong as that in the kleptomaniac or suicidal monomaniac. The degeneration of simple inebriety into pure accepted forms of lunacy, and the frequent history of insanity in the progenitors of inebriates, are evidences which strongly support an opinion the result of clinical observation.'

An habitual drunkard may now also be dealt with under the Act for the Prevention of Cruelty to Children 1894, if he or she is the parent of the child, or is living with the parent of the child, and is convicted of any of the following offences: (1) cruelty to children within the meaning of the Act; (2) neglect or refusal to provide necessary food, clothing, or lodging to an apprentice or servant, doing them bodily harm, so as to endanger life or health; (3) causing a child to take part in any public exhibition or performance whereby, in the opinion of a court of summary jurisdiction, the life or limbs of such child shall be endangered; or (4) committing any other offence involving bodily injury to a child under the age of 16 years.[1] Upon conviction for any of these offences, the court, in lieu of sentencing such person to imprisonment, may order his detention for any period not exceeding twelve months in a retreat, and the order is to have the same effect as an application made and approved under the Habitual Drunkards Acts. But there are three conditions: (1) the person, having had such notice as the court deems sufficient of the intention to allege habitual drunkenness, must consent to have the order made; (2) any representations of the wife or husband, objecting to the order being made, must be taken into consideration; and (3) 'before making the order the court shall, to such extent as it may seem reasonably sufficient, be satisfied that provision will be made for defraying the expenses of such person during detention in a retreat.'

XXI.—DISCHARGED PRISONERS.

For the aid of discharged prisoners there is more than one Society in London. In the course of the year one or two cases of this kind will probably come under the almoner's attention. Prisoners' Aid Societies are 'certified' by Justices in quarter sessions.[2] To aid prisoners on their discharge a certain sum, voted annually by the Government, is apportioned to each prisoner according to the annual discharges. This apportionment the Societies receive under certain restrictions, to be applied for the prisoners' benefit; but a sum exceeding £2, inclusive of 'mark' money, cannot be expended on any one prisoner.[3]

Certified Prisoners' Aid Societies.

Allowances to discharged prisoners.

XXII.—VAGRANTS, CASUALS, AND HOMELESS CASES.

To give money in the streets to beggars, and do nothing more, is, in the eyes of charity, a crime. People say, if I have relieved one deserving case out of ten to whom I have given money, I have done a good work. But, first, nine may have been injured on that hypothesis, and nine persons so relieved must almost certainly be injured; next, the dole has relieved one person, but no one can be relieved properly

Giving alms in the streets.

---

[1] Prevention of Cruelty to Children Act 1894, 57 & 58 Vict., c. 41, s. 11, and schedule referring to the Offences against the Person Act 1861, 24 & 25 Vict., c. 100, and the Children's Dangerous Performance Act, 42 & 43 Vict., c. 34.

[2] 25 & 26 Vict., c. 44, s. 1.

[3] *See* letter of Home Secretary to the Chairmen of Discharged Prisoners' Aid Societies, 5 March, 1880.

by a dole; then, again, the ten gifts represented ten seductive chances to poor persons, who have little inducement enough, apart from such bribes as these, to stick to their work; and, lastly, 'deserving,' the favourite word of thoughtless almsgivers, implies a wrong test. Strictly used, it is merciless; loosely used it is meaningless. Almoners should assist in order to cure and not in order to reward.

What to do when asked for charity in the streets.

A person who asks alms of a stranger may be referred by him to a casual ward or to a Charity Organisation Committee. If the case is of such a kind as is *primâ facie* unsuitable for reference to the casual ward, the Committee would give whatever immediate help may be required, and finally deal with it after inquiry. There is no room for doubting that the applications in the streets are in almost every instance made by indolent persons, who live sometimes in and sometimes out of the workhouse, and are seldom engaged in hard work of any kind. To refer them to those who will look into their circumstances may be wise; but to give them money (or food) is to invest it in manufacturing pauperism.

The Poor Law arrangements for the casual poor or pauper.

The 'casual poor are those poor persons who are not settled in the parish or reside there, but who happen casually to be there at the time when, from some accident occurring to them, or being suddenly afflicted with some illness, they are obliged to resort to the parish officer for relief.'[1] For the care of these casual poor, if they be admitted into the workhouse, the General Order (Consolidated), July 24, 1847, provides. But the casual poor are chiefly 'destitute wayfarers or wanderers applying for and receiving relief,' and, under the title of 'casual paupers,' special provision has been made for them since that date by way of 'casual wards.' For their convenience there are casual wards—proper sleeping accommodation, consisting of separate cells, beds, and compartments, or other arrangements approved by the Local Government Board. There is a fixed dietary and scale of task work, to be done by the casual in return for the food and lodging. In the metropolis the wards are inspected, on behalf of the Local Government Board, once in every four months. They are open to casuals between October and March inclusive after 6 P.M., between April and September after 8 P.M. Orders, which are available only for the night for which they are issued,[2] are given by a relieving officer, or, in cases of sudden and urgent necessity, by an overseer; but the master of the workhouse or superintendent of a casual ward may admit without order cases of urgent necessity, or, if there is room in the ward, persons brought to it by a constable. Refusals to admit them are to be reported to the Guardians. Any policeman in the metropolis may conduct any destitute wayfarer, wanderer, or foundling, or

---

[1] Glen's Archbold, p. 281.
[2] Pauper Inmates' Discharge and Regulation Act (34 & 35 Vict., c. 108).

other destitute person, to a casual ward personally.[1] On his admission every casual is searched; all articles found on him are taken from him and returned on his discharge, except money, which is retained. He has to take a bath; he is supplied with other clothes while in the ward; his own are dried, disinfected, and returned to him on leaving. The casual is liable, on conviction, to hard labour for one month as 'idle and disorderly' (see p. lxvi.), if he abscond, refuse or neglect to do his work, or fail to observe the regulations; or if he wilfully gives a false name or makes a false statement for the purpose of obtaining relief. And if, besides committing these offences, he has on a previous occasion been convicted as 'an idle and disorderly person,' or if he destroys his own clothes, or the Guardians' property, he is punished as a 'rogue and a vagabond' (see p. lxvi.). The master of the workhouse can take a disorderly inmate or casual before the magistrate without warrant.[2]

Subject to discretionary power in the hands of the Guardians, a casual pauper cannot discharge himself before 9 o'clock in the morning of the day following his admission, nor before he has performed the work prescribed for him. If he has already been admitted once in the period of a month to any of the casual wards in the metropolis, he is not entitled to discharge himself before 9 A.M. on the fourth day after his admission, and he may during that interval be removed to the workhouse. Sunday is not included in the computation of days.[3]

But discretion in regard to the application of this rule is vested in the Guardians and their officers :—

'(1) The Guardians may give any directions to the master of the workhouse, or to the superintendent of the casual ward, with respect to the discharge of any class or classes of casual paupers before the expiration of the respective periods specified in the section above cited, and such directions shall be followed by the master or superintendent;

'(2) If, in the opinion of the master of the workhouse, or the superintendent of the casual ward, any special circumstances shall require that a casual pauper shall be discharged before the expiration of the periods mentioned, . . . he may discharge such pauper accordingly, and report the facts of the case to the Guardians at their next meeting.

'(3) A casual pauper who has been detained for more than one night, and who represents to the master of the workhouse or the superintendent of the casual ward that he is desirous of seeking work, shall, if he has to the best of his ability performed the prescribed task of work, be allowed to discharge himself at the time hereinafter mentioned on the day upon which he is discharged; that is to say —

'During the period between Lady-Day and Michaelmas-Day . . . half-past five o'clock in the morning;

'During the period between Michaelmas-Day and Lady-Day . . . half-past six o'clock in the morning.

'The request of such casual pauper shall not be refused except on the ground

---

[1] Metropolitan Houseless Poor Act, sec 4. As a rule, all cases of real or apparent urgency in the streets should be brought to the notice of the police, or referred or taken to a workhouse or casual ward.

[2] 34 & 35 Vict., c. 108, s. 8.   [3] Casual Poor Act 1882 (44 & 45 Vict., c. 36).

that he has not performed the prescribed task of work to the best of his ability,
and every such refusal shall be reported to the Guardians at their next ordinary
meeting. by the master of the workhouse or the superintendent of the casual ward,
as the case may be.'[1]

There is thus free public accommodation for all travellers
who, being without money, are prepared to put up with rather
rough accommodation, and to do a task of work by way of payment. This provision, unless carefully guarded, has a tendency to
harbour vagrants and to facilitate vagrancy. Especially is this
the case where the wards are 'associated,' and the men can
gossip and compare notes and settle plans with one another. But
wards consisting of separate cells, both for sleeping and for
performing the task, are now being introduced; and these,
provided the full task of an ordinary nine hours' day be required,
appear to reduce vagrancy. For the ordinary vagrant, and for that
class of wanderers who profess that they are not vagrants, but are
men who are unemployed and are seeking work, this system is suitable. For those 'undoubted working men making their way as
quickly as they can from one centre of industry to another to work
which they know to be awaiting them,'[2] generally speaking no
provision is necessary. But if they do require casual relief, they
would undoubtedly prefer the 'separate' to the 'associated' system.

Obligations
of the
charitable. Upon the charitable in regard to vagrants, two chief obligations
are laid: As a rule to refuse relief, but to inquire into and to try to
assist thoroughly any cases in which—judging from a knowledge of
the class—it may seem likely that the vagrant, tramp, or wanderer
may be placed in self-dependence. With the young especially this
is sometimes possible. The following is an instance of apparent
success :—

'F. P. is a boy of 17, pock-marked, and starved in appearance. Some years ago
his father deserted him, and for eighteen months he had been in the workhouse
school. From there he was placed in the House Boy Brigade, and transferred
immediately to a working boys' home. He said that there he was sent out to
get work, but could not succeed on account of deficient eyesight, and that, afraid
of being unable to pay his expenses at the home, he ran away, and tramped about
homeless for three or four months, when he was found in a London casual ward.
The character given him rom his former school was not good. This boy was
placed in the Lads' Labour Home in the neighbourhood, where for the last five
weeks he has earned his living by wood-chopping. Clothes were given him. He
has now obtained an indoor situation as sorter in a shop at Battersea.'

This, on the other hand, is a case of apparent failure :—

'M. R. was a helpless and hopeless looking girl over 18. Admission was
obtained for her from a casual ward to a home. and then she was transferred to a
hospital. She could not be received back at the home, as her conduct had been
bad whilst in it. But it was ascertained that she had good parents and a good

[1] Order Amending General Order ('Regulations as to Casual Paupers'),
18 December, 1882: Annual Report: Local Government Board, 1892-3, p. 14.
[2] See a paper on Vagrancy, with reference to the effect of the Act of 1882, by
Mr. W. E. Knollys, Local Government Inspector.

home of her own in the North of London. She was therefore returned to it, but there is some reason to believe she has run away again, and probably will reappear at the casual ward.'[1]

It will again and again be noticed how many 'chances' those who sink into the vagrant class have had—how often their friends, and then charitable persons outside their family, have helped them, found them employment, forgiven them, and tried to make the best of them. Thorough assistance in this branch of work is most difficult. If children, as in the cases above quoted, have been so often relieved and aided without good result, the task of helping the adult is, it will be realised, still more difficult and often quite hopeless. Generally speaking, there is only one method, and that will, after all, rescue only a small percentage—the alliance for mutual help and assistance of the almoner and charity with the Guardians and the Poor Law, the provision of some means, as in F. P.'s case, of test and supervision. The latter may be as practicable, with the help of a good workhouse master, in a workhouse as in any other institution. The individual by himself, however earnest he may be, cannot accomplish much without the organised and systematic assistance of others. But for work of this kind no further supply of charitable refuges or shelters is wanted. These are usually planned on the 'associated' principle, and are often without the bath and the other salutary and sanitary contrivances of the casual ward. At the casual wards there is an ample field for charitable intervention under at least as good conditions. Whoever wishes to do this work should turn them to account.

The other obligation which is imposed upon the charitable is to promote uniformity in the general methods of dealing with vagrancy. The number of vagrants in relation to the population is not large. The mean number relieved (1st January and 1st July) 1893 in England and Wales was 6,888.[2] Of those who obtained relief, about 75 per cent. probably are recurrent cases.[3] A night census of homeless persons in refuges and casual wards in London on January 19, 1891, showed the total to be 1,781. A night census of tramps and vagrants, both in casual wards and common lodging houses, in Wiltshire showed that their number in that county was 79 on December 1, 1892; 101 on December 1, 1893. In Gloucestershire a similar census, taken annually on the first Tuesday in April, proves that their numbers have varied since 1887 only from 74 to 103. Usually about half of those included in the census are, it is stated, living entirely by tramping. In Scotland the night census of vagrants in prisons or police cells, refuges and poor-houses, common lodging and other houses, public parks, outhouses, &c., on June 26, 1892, gave the following figures: 6,027, or 63 per cent., adult males; 2,042, or

---

[1] 'Some Cases from Casual Wards,' *Charity Organisation Review*, January 1892.
[2] Local Government Board Report, p. 269.
[3] *Cf.* 'Vagrancy,' a paper by Mr. G. Paul, Workhouse Master at Knaresborough, Poor Law Conferences, 1892.

21 per cent., adult females ; 1,486, or 16 per cent., children under 14. The vagrants numbered 1·59 per thousand of the population. Finally, Colonel Curtis Hayward estimates the number of vagrants at not more than 10,000.[1] The number no doubt rises and falls, to some extent, according to the industrial condition of the country. In bad times a certain number of unskilled labourers tramp after work, who in good times remain settled and employed. But, after making every allowance, the total number is not very large, and it would seem quite possible to limit it still further by the adoption of a uniform system.

A Special Committee of the Charity Organisation Society on the Homeless Poor of London made the following recommendations in 1891.   They deal especially with London :—

SUMMARY OF THE PRINCIPAL RECOMMENDATIONS OF THE COMMITTEE.

1. It seems clear that the accommodation in the casual wards and the refuges mentioned in the Report is more than sufficient to meet the demand. The total accommodation is for 2,896 persons: the inmates on January 16, 1891, were only 1,781. Thus it appears that no further shelters, pure and simple, are required.

2. The Committee would strongly recommend that some of the existing accommodation should be used for the purpose of small homes for the careful treatment, from a religious and moral point of view, of individuals who, it is thought, may be reclaimed.

3. It is obvious that, as a matter of humanity, every destitute person, good, bad, or indifferent, ought to have the opportunity of obtaining a night's shelter in London ; but the Committee are strongly of opinion that all vagrants and homeless persons who seem incapable of being reclaimed and raised from their position of dependence should be left to the Poor Law, to be received either in the workhouses or the casual wards, and that the charitable refuges should deal with the helpable only, treating each case according to its particular requirements, and endeavouring to bring back the their sympathetic care to a settled mode of life, thus diminishing homelessness instead of merely relieving and thereby encouraging it.

4. In the opinion of the Committee investigation should, as soon as possible, be made into the condition and antecedents of each applicant for admission to a refuge, with the object of ascertaining whether he can be helped, and what form of assistance is most appropriate to his case. Pending investigation, the applicant should either be received provisionally into the refuge or sent on to the casual ward or workhouse.

5. It would seem unwise to fix any period for the ordinary duration of stay at the refuges ; the period should rather be adapted to the circumstances of the individual case. Similarly it is, in the opinion of the Committee, inexpedient to make a rule of refusing readmission within a certain time: the question should depend upon the reason in the particular case for readmission becoming needful.

6. The Committee are of opinion that the casual ward system should be amended. They think that greatly increased powers of detention, in regard to habitual or recurrent cases, should be given, and, while retaining the casual wards for the reception of casual paupers in the first instance, they would suggest that, where the increased powers of detention are exercised, the pauper should be sent on to the workhouse to complete his period of detention, being treated there somewhat less favourably than the resident pauper as regards diet or otherwise, and subjected to a system of 'dissociation,' and industrial occupation, such as Mr. Vallance recommends.

7. In the opinion of the Committee no real improvement in the condition of the homeless can be effected except by co-operation between the Poor Law and

---

[1] West Midland Poor Law Conference, 1894.

charity, and between the various charitable institutions *inter se*. And, for this purpose, the Committee recommend that each refuge should link itself with a certain number of casual wards, the Guardians being asked to give the superintendents of their wards power to send on to the refuge persons who might appear helpable. In the event of the Council suggested below being established, such arrangements might best be brought about by consultation with that body. The Committee recommend the formation of a Council for the purposes of organisation and consultation, consisting of Poor Law Guardians, representatives of refuges, and others interested in the homeless class. The work of such a Council would be:

(1) To arrange with Guardians for a systematic visitation of the various casual wards, with the object of picking out helpable cases and referring them to appropriate charitable institutions.

(2) To secure the proper investigation and treatment of homeless cases.

(3) To arrange for the inspection of refuges on the lines of the existing inspection of casual wards, for the purpose of detecting ineligible persons, and so preventing them from resorting successively to the various refuges. To employ one or more inspectors for a similar purpose.

8. The Committee would also have had much pleasure in making some recommendations for the benefit of old soldiers, who are found in such large numbers amongst the homeless class, and they cannot but feel that there must be something radically wrong in the short service system which compels men with good discharges to seek the aid of the charitable public. The question, however, is such a large one, and of so great importance, that it can only be dealt with by the authorities at the War Office, who, the Committee understand, are now considering the question.

In the country uniformity of provision for vagrants is quite as important as it is in London. At present often the vagrants are not detained for the second night. If they are numerous the ward cannot receive them all, and they have to be sent on to the relieving officer, who gives them a ticket to a common lodging house. There is in these cases no task of work at all; and in others the task of work is wholly insufficient. The safeguards which the law requires for the prevention of vagrancy are thus neglected, and a system, which is serviceable enough when properly carried out, breaks down because conditions essential to its success are not uniformly adopted.

Outside the workhouse or casual ward there is the same need of uniformity—on the part of almsgivers. The sparrows will come where every day breadcrumbs are thrown to them, so will the vagrants resort wherever houses good for their purpose are to be found; and, moreover, in the country it is a matter of common knowledge that they are often relieved out of fear of their threats rather than out of sympathy for their condition. As a substitute for the casual relief which they obtain at houses and cottages, endeavour is made in several counties to supply them with absolute necessaries, such as bread, in such a way that the almsgiver may at least feel that they need not starve, and that, being sufficiently provided for, they do not require his help. The Dorsetshire and Gloucestershire systems have, both alike, this object. By the latter way, tickets are supplied under the supervision of the

e

police: and the vagrant that keeps to his route has preferential treatment : and to meet his actual needs bread is supplied. By the former, the Dorsetshire system, tickets for bread are widely distributed to residents throughout the county: the tickets are exchangeable for bread at certain shops on the main roads, and however large the number of tickets the vagrant may have in his possession, he can only be supplied with a fixed amount of bread in return for them. The object of both these methods is to make the public understand that, as the needs of the vagrants are fully met by the Poor Law and by the bread tickets, the vagrants cannot be in want, and may therefore be refused relief. The success of both methods depends largely on constant propagandism in the country.

Poor Law provision for cases of sudden and urgent necessity.

In addition to the system of casual wards, there are stringent legal provisions for the assistance of cases 'of sudden and urgent necessity.' In such cases the relieving officer has to afford relief either by admission to the workhouse, or by relief (not in money) out of the workhouse. The powers of the masters of workhouses and of the police in such cases we have alluded to (*see* p. xlii.). In any case of sickness or accident, requiring medical attendance, the relieving officer has to give an order on the district medical officer. The cost of relief given in cases of accident or sudden illness is paid by the Union in which application is made, subject to reimbursement from the Union to which the applicant belongs. Justices of the Peace may give an order for medical relief [1] in cases of sudden and dangerous illness, irrespective of settlement.

XXIII.—STREET BEGGARS AND VAGABONDS.

Laws regarding begging, etc.

We pass from the casual and vagrant poor to the law for punishment of idle and disorderly persons and rogues and vagabonds 'in that part of Great Britain called England.' [2]

There are—

(1) Idle and disorderly persons.

(2) Rogues and vagabonds.

(3) Incorrigible rogues and vagabonds.

In the first category comes 'every person wandering abroad, or placing himself or herself in any public place, street, highway, court, or passage, to beg or gather alms, or causing, or procuring, or encouraging any child or children (under 16) to do so.' The punishment for this is hard labour for any time not exceeding one calendar month. [3] The offender can be convicted if the

[1] 4 Will. IV., c. 76, s. 54.   [2] 5 Geo. IV., c. 83, s. 3. etc.
[3] In lieu of imprisonment fines may be required in accordance with the scale in the Summary Jurisdiction Act 1879, in the case of idle and disorderly persons, and rogues and vagabonds. The provisions of this Act so far as it concerns children have been greatly strengthened by the Prevention of Cruelty to Children Act 1894 (*see* p. xcix.).

Justice saw the offence committed, if the offender confesses, or if one or more credible witnesses give evidence against the offender on oath.

In the second category comes 'every person committing any of the offences hereinbefore mentioned *after* having been convicted as an idle and disorderly person . . . every person wandering abroad and endeavouring, by the exposure of wounds or deformities, to obtain or gather alms, or endeavouring to procure charitable contributions of any nature or kind, under any false or fraudulent pretence.' The punishment in this case is hard labour for not more than three months. Conviction is by confession or on evidence on oath (as above).

In the third category is placed 'every person committing an offence against this Act which shall subject him or her to be dealt with as a rogue and vagabond, such person having been at some former time adjudged so to be and duly convicted thereof.'

The punishment is in this case committal to the House of Correction with hard labour till the next general or quarter sessions; and at quarter sessions the incorrigible rogue may be further imprisoned with hard labour for one year, and (if not a female) punished by whipping.

It should be noted that it is lawful for any person whatsoever to apprehend anyone 'found offending against this Act,' and forthwith to take him, or cause a constable to take him, before a Justice.[1] A constable is liable to a penalty of 5*l.* if he refuses or wilfully neglects to take such a person into custody, or does not use his best endeavours to apprehend and convey him before a Justice. There, by the Justice's order, he may be searched; and on conviction money found on him is applied to the expenses of his apprehension and maintenance. On warrant lodging-houses suspected of concealing vagrants and persons of the above classes can be searched by the police or other persons.

XXIV.— BEGGING-LETTER WRITERS.

'False or fraudulent pretence,' in the second category of offences just mentioned, suggests 'begging-letter writers.' The habit of begging naturally leads to the exaggeration of facts, often true and pitiable, which become the beggar's stock-in-trade. The habit of responding to begging-letters leads to the encouragement of this form of lying. The fault is with both beggar and giver. Instead of ascertaining and considering the facts, and assisting accordingly, the donor gives as a quittance a contribution,

---

[1] This Act, besides the offences mentioned in the above categories, deals with, amongst others, cases of persons wilfully refusing to maintain themselves and their families (*see* p. lii.). In these cases also, therefore, any person may take the initiative.

which is probably spent by the recipient in immediate needs, if not turned to evil uses. The one lacks charity and gives money; the other learns the lesson of begging, and makes money out of charity. The only remedy is to inquire, and, in eligible cases, to help thoroughly. Repressive measures, prosecutions, and the like, can only open people's eyes to the need of inquiry. In themselves they are useless. If donors were not the prey of piteous tales, and roused to give rather by a show of words than by a knowledge of facts, it might be said that the money given to worthless beggars was money of which those in distress were robbed. But now this money seems their fair spoil; at least they are more entitled to it than the donors who give it away without thinking that its worth is only in its suitable application; and the distressed have practically no chance of obtaining it, for distress cannot compete successfully with practised hypocrisy.

'False pretences.'

Penal servitude for five years, or imprisonment for two, is the punishment of anyone who is convicted of having by false pretence obtained from any person any chattel, money, or valuable security, with intent to defraud.[1] Anyone may apprehend and take before a Justice, without warrant, a person *found committing* this offence. 'There must be (1) an intentional and specific statement of some pretended *existing fact* which the maker knows to be untrue; (2) it must be material to the matter in hand; (3) it must be made with intent to defraud; and (4) the person to whom it is addressed must, in point of fact, believe it, and make over property on the strength of it.'[2] The attempt to obtain property by false pretences is indictable.

Mendicant charitable institutions.

Many so-called charities exist by begging of strangers. Much of this begging is carried on by letter and circular; much by a house-to-house visitation of those who seem likely to be able to spare a little for a charitable purpose. Agents call at houses in the suburbs, and tell of spiritual destitution and want. The master of the house is absent. They are asked no questions; they show a collection-book and a list of donors, and, possibly, of members of committee. No word they say is verified. They receive countless small donations, and their profits are large. From beginning to end, except perhaps in that wish to do good which makes the listener feel in his pocket for a half-crown, there is not a jot of charity in the whole transaction. Here, again, inquiry is the only remedy. Donors have to learn to support only useful and well-regulated charitable institutions, which give on inquiry good guarantees for their work and management.

One of the prevalent forms of mendicity in the Metropolis is

[1] 24 & 25 Vict., c. 96, s. 88.
[2] 'The Justice's Note Book,' by W. Knox Wigram, p. 204.

worthy of mention. It is that of Volunteer Fire Brigades, Volunteer
Fire
Brigades
in the
Metropolis. which, with hardly an exception, are conducted for the personal benefit of one or two promoters, and are quite useless for extinguishing fires. Their collectors appear in the dress of firemen, and the unwary may be led to believe that they are men of the Metropolitan Brigade. The responsibility of 'providing and maintaining an efficient force of firemen, and of furnishing them with all such fire-engines, horses, accoutrements, tools, and implements for the complete equipment of the force, or conducive to the efficient performance of their duties,' rests with the London County Council.[1] With regard to Volunteer Brigades it is enacted ' that on the occasion of a fire the chief or other officer in charge of any fire brigade may, on his discretion, take the command of any volunteer fire brigade.' These brigades therefore have a *locus standi*, such as it is; and it is argued that the provision made by the Council for several of the outlying parts of the Metropolis is insufficient. On the latter point there may be some ground of complaint. The expenses of the Brigade are met by contributions from Fire Insurance Companies, and by a rate of a halfpenny in the pound in the Metropolis. The sum at the disposal of the Council from these sources is insufficient, and Bills have been introduced into Parliament for increasing it, hitherto without result. But even if this hindrance be removed, the Volunteer Brigades are likely to remain. They are a source of profit to their proprietors, though useless for real service. If, therefore, they are to be recognised at all, some system of licenses is necessary. The licenses might be granted by the County Council and the Police, and it might be made an offence for any unlicensed brigade to collect contributions. The evil would then be checked.

The Metropolitan Fire Brigade never sends men from house to house to collect subscriptions. All such applications by, or on behalf of, firemen should be summarily rejected.

XXV.—Pedlars.

The pedlar is a kind of legalised vagrant— a vagrant with a Cost of
pedlar's cer-
tificate, etc. 'legitimate and recognised purpose in roving. Almoners will often have applications made to them to ' renew stock ' and to pay for a pedlar's certificate. The words pedlar and hawker are often used indifferently. Hawker is the name of the genus, with two species, one also named ' hawker ' and one ' pedlar.' Both hawker and pedlar, when provided with license or certificate, are ' licensed hawkers '; but the hawker takes out a license, for which he pays £4, and ' pursues his hawking trade on horseback or inside his caravan,' and carries to sell or expose to sale ' goods to be afterwards

<hr>

[1] Metropolitan Fire Brigade Act, 28 & 29 Vict., cap. 90 (1865).

delivered,' while the pedlar 'travels or trades on foot' without any horse or other beast bearing or drawing burden, and sells goods 'to be immediately delivered, or offers for sale his skill in handicraft,' and has to take out a yearly certificate, for which he pays 5s. It is with him rather than with the hawker that the almoner will come in contact. He obtains his certificate from the chief office of the police district in which he resides. Any policeman may open and inspect his pack; and if he resists or has no certificate, he may be apprehended. If convicted of begging, the magistrate has to deprive him of his certificate; if convicted of other offences under the Act (34 & 35 Vict., c. 96), each offence has to be endorsed on the certificate. Many itinerant persons profess to be licensed hawkers; if they allege that they are in distress, it is always well to ask for their certificate. Hawkers' licenses are not required for the sale of printed papers 'licensed by authority,' fish, fruit, or vegetables, nor for the sale of goods by their makers or the maker's servants. Nor are licenses required of tinkers, harness-menders, and others who carry about with them materials for mending household goods; nor for 'people who are makers of their goods or wares, or servants of such makers; wholesale traders; and persons selling coals by retail.'[1]

XXVI.—Soldiers and Seamen: their Liabilities and Means of Providing for their Families during Absence, etc.

For another class, whose work takes them from home, the law makes special provision. Many cases occur in which the almoner may want information in regard to the liability of the soldier or seaman to support his family; the possibility of his assigning his pay, or making out an allotment for their benefit. In this section these points are touched on in regard to (1) Soldiers, Seamen and Marines in the Royal Navy, and (2) Seamen in the Merchant Service.

1.—Soldiers; Seamen and Marines in the Royal Navy.

Soldiers and sailors appear to be liable, like other men, to support their kindred, but it is not always easy to enforce the liability.

The following enactments may be noticed:—

Soldiers.

1. Soldiers serving in the regular forces are not personally amenable to the civil courts, excepting (1) on account of a charge or conviction for crime, (2) on account of any debt or damages or sum of money, when the amount sought to be recovered exceeds £30 over and above all costs of suit.[2] A soldier, however, may,

[1] See 'The Justice's Note Book,' pp. 238 and 350. 50 Geo. III., c. 41, s. 16,; 22 & 23 Vict., c. 36 s. 3; 24 & 25 Vict., c. 21, s. 9.

[2] Army Act 1881, 44 & 45 Vict., c. 58, s. 144.

after notice in writing, be sued to judgment in the ordinary course, but is protected from the issue of execution against his person, pay, arms, or clothing.[1]

Indeed, it seems that his pay cannot be touched in any way except under a special provision, by which he is declared to be liable to contribute to the maintenance of his wife and children and of any bastard child to the same extent as if he were not a soldier.[2] This liability, which specifically includes the cost of any relief given to his wife or child by way of loan, is enforced by sending a copy of the order or decree establishing it to a Secretary of State, who thereupon is bound to order a portion of his daily pay, not exceeding 6d. in the case of a non-commissioned officer who is not below the rank of sergeant, and 3d. in the case of any other soldier, to be stopped, to meet the claim.[3]

Furthermore, if it be shown to the satisfaction of the Secretary of State that a soldier serving in the regular forces has deserted or left in destitute circumstances without reasonable cause his wife or any of his legitimate children under 14 years of age, the Secretary has to withhold his pay in a similar manner, and apply it towards the maintenance of the wife or children in such manner as he may think fit.[4]

A soldier is ' not liable to be *punished* for the offence of deserting or neglecting his wife and family, or leaving them chargeable to the rates.'[5]

2. As regards Reserve men and pensioners, we find that no military pay, reward, or pension is capable of assignment by the soldier to his widow, child, or other relative who may be entitled to it, except in pursuance of a Royal Warrant for the benefit of the family of the person entitled to it, or under an Act of Parliament.[6]

Reserve men and Pensioners : Pay, etc., not assignable.

3. If First-class Army Reserve men are called out, they receive an allowance from the Government of 8d. a day for their wives and 2d. a day for each girl under 16 or boy under 14. This allowance is issued monthly, in advance. Guardians, if applications are made to them to assist the families of reserve men, have to decide ' whether the applicants are really destitute to such an extent as to require relief.' The pay and allowances of men are such that, ' as a rule, an able-bodied woman should have no difficulty in finding, if not immediately, at least within a reasonable period of her husband's departure, sufficient employment to enable her to maintain

Assistance to wives of Army Reserve when called out.

---

[1] Army Act 1881, 44 & 45 Vict., c. 58, s. 136.

[2] Ibid., s. 145.

[3] 46 & 47 Vict., c. 6, s. 7.

[4] 177th Article of War. Cf. Glen, p. 228.

[5] Army Act 1881 (44 & 45 Vict., c. 58). Cf. Archbold, p. 334, and *supra*, p. lii.

[6] Ibid., s. 141.

adequately herself and her children, if any.' Only temporary help at the utmost should therefore be required, and, 'where the applications are made for the first time, and the Guardians are quite satisfied that some assistance is necessary, outdoor relief may not improperly be granted for a short period, in order to enable the applicants to make such arrangements for their support as their altered circumstances may really require.'[1]

Claim on military and naval pensions of persons relieved from the rates.

4. Next as regards military and naval pensioners :—

(1) When relief by admission to the workhouse has been given by the Guardians to any person entitled to any army or navy pension or any superannuation or other allowance, or to his wife, or to any person whom he may be liable to maintain. In this case he may transmit to the Paymaster-General a minute according to a form provided by the Act,[2] requiring that the next quarter's pension be paid to them.

(2) When any such person, entitled to a pension, applies for temporary relief to a Board of Guardians, it shall be lawful ' but not compulsory on their part ' to require the pensioner to assign to them[3] his next quarterly payment of pension.

(3) If a Chelsea or Greenwich out-pensioner or his family becomes chargeable,[4] the Secretary of State may agree with the Guardians for repayment out of the pension, provided that, if relief has been given to the wife and one child only, not more than one-half of the pension, or, if relief has been given to two or more children, or to the wife and one or more children, not more than two-thirds of the pension be appropriated. ' If the pensioner and his family be relieved in the workhouse, the Guardians have no legal right to, and cannot claim any larger amount of, the pension than is equivalent to the actual cost of the paupers in the workhouse.'[5]

It should be noted, however, that ' the Lords Commissioners of the Admiralty say that the Act of Parliament which authorises Guardians to receive pensions, does not apply to Greenwich Hospital or service pensions, which will in future be paid to the pensioners themselves, although they may be inmates of workhouses, or in receipt of outdoor relief.'[6]

Seamen in Royal Navy and Marines.

As regards seamen in the Royal Navy and Marines, it may be noticed :—

1. Assignments of naval pay and pensions are void.[7]

2. Seamen and marines serving under the Naval Discipline Act are not liable to be arrested in respect of any debt contracted

---

[1] Local Government Board Circular, August 30, 1882.
[2] 2 & 3 Vict., c. 51, s. 2.   [3] Ibid., s. 3.
[4] 19 Vict., c. 15, ss. 8 and 9.   [5] Glen, p. 446.
[6] Ibid., p. 427.
[7] The Naval and Marine Pay and Pensions Act 1865, 28 & 29 Vict., c. 73, ss. 4 and 5.

while the debtor belonged to the Queen's Service.[1] They are, however, liable to arrest while in the United Kingdom as a means of enforcing the following orders[2] :—

(1) An affiliation order, under 35 & 36 Vict., c. 65, s. 4 (*see* p. liii.).

(2) An order on a husband, convicted of an aggravated assault upon his wife, to pay her a weekly sum, under 41 & 42 Vict., c. 19, s. 4 (*see* p. lxxxviii.).

(3) An order on a husband, who has deserted his wife, to pay her a weekly sum, under 49 & 50 Vict., c. 52, s. 1 (*see* p. lxxxvii.).

(4) An order, made by a competent court, at the instance of Guardians, for the cost of relief supplied to persons whom he is bound to support.

3. The Admiralty has no power to make any deduction from a seaman's pay for the support of his wife, family, or bastard child while he is afloat; he is then serving under the Naval Discipline Act.[3] Captains and officers are, however, instructed to use their influence with the men to encourage them to make due provision for the support of their wives and families; and if the wife makes a complaint to the Admiralty that her husband has left her destitute, and supports her statement by the certificate of any magistrate or minister of religion, her application will for this purpose be referred to the captain under whom the husband is serving, with a view to his inducing the man to allot.

When serving on shore marines are under the Army Act, and can be placed under stoppage for the support of their wives, families, or bastard children.

4. Seamen and marines may make allotments of their full pay at the higher or other rates specified in the regulations in favour of any persons over the age of 18 years, or to a trustee for a person below that age. Allotments of pay.

Boys, after six months' service, may, if they keep their clothes in order, allot in favour of a father, or mother, or the Naval Savings Bank, or if orphans to the guardians by whom they were brought up. First class boys can send home 8s., second class 6s. a week.

The allotment note here referred to is a document stating that as A.B., serving on board H.M. ship............, has made an allotment of his pay to C.D., the Paymaster-General, or other responsible officer as specified, is required to allot a sum mentioned, month by month, subject to the production of a formal certificate of the allottee's identity by a magistrate or minister. Payment must be demanded within six months; and the note, if not previously stopped, holds

---

[1] 29 & 30 Vict., c. 109, s. 97.　　[2] 29 & 30 Vict., c. 109, s. 101.
[3] *See* Regulations of 1893, Article 1,664, etc.

good for four years. The allotment note may be made payable at any Post Office.

II.—*Seamen in the Merchant Service.*

As regards seamen in the merchant service, we find the following provisions in the Merchant Shipping Act, 57 & 58 Vict., c. 60, which consolidated the enactments on this subject:—

1. 'Any stipulation made by a seaman at the commencement of a voyage for the allotment of any part of his wages during his absence has to be inserted in the agreement with the crew, and must state the amounts and times of the payments to be made. Where the agreement is required to be made in a form approved by the Board of Trade, the seaman may require that a stipulation be inserted in the agreement for the allotment, by means of an allotment note, of any part (not exceeding one-half) of his wages in favour either of a near relative or a savings bank.' By a 'near relative' is meant a wife, father, mother, grandfather, grandmother, child, grandchild, brother, or sister. The shipowner or any agent who has authorised the drawing of the note is liable upon it, and may be sued by the person in whose favour it is drawn in the county court or summarily before justices of the peace. In any such proceeding the seaman is presumed to be duly earning his wages unless the contrary be shown. A wife who deserts her children or so misconducts herself as to be undeserving of support from her husband forfeits her right to further payments under an allotment note.

Allotment notes must be in a form approved by the Board of Trade. 'A payment under an allotment note shall begin at the expiration of one month, or, if the allotment is in favour of a savings bank, of three months from the date of the agreement with the crew, or at such later date as may be fixed by the agreement, and shall be paid at the expiration of every subsequent month, or of such other periods as may be fixed by the agreement, and shall be paid only in respect of wages earned before the date of payment.'

2. In addition to the system of allotment notes there are abundant facilities given to seamen to save their wages or other money by means of seamen's savings banks established under the Board of Trade in the principal ports in the United Kingdom, and to transmit money to their relatives or other persons by money orders to be obtained at the mercantile marine offices.

3. If the wife, children, or stepchildren of a seaman become chargeable to the Union during his absence on a voyage, the Union is entitled to be reimbursed to the extent of half his wages if one such relation, and two-thirds if two or more such relations, be

chargeable ; but the claim of the Union is diminished by any sum paid by the owner of the ship under an allotment note in their favour.

The Guardians may give a notice in writing to the owner of the ship stating the proportion of the seaman's wages upon which they propose to make a claim, and the owner thereupon is bound to retain in hand the amount for a period of twenty-one days after the seaman's return to his port of discharge, and on his return give him notice of their intended claim. On the application of the Guardians, a court of summary jurisdiction may ' make a summary order for the reimbursement to the whole extent claimed, or to such lesser extent as the court, under the circumstances, think fit ; and the owner shall pay to the Board or inspector out of the seaman's wages the amount so ordered to be paid by way of reimbursement, and shall pay the residue of the wages to the seaman. If no order for reimbursement is obtained within the period mentioned in the notice given to the owner as aforesaid, the proportion of wages to be retained by him shall immediately on the expiration of that period, and without deduction, be payable to the seaman.'

4. The law has imposed upon the owners of ships the duty of providing medical treatment and subsistence for the seamen who are hurt or fall ill in their service.

5. ' The Board of Trade ' ' make regulations with respect to the relief, maintenance, and sending home of seamen and apprentices found in distress abroad.' ' (a) Seamen and apprentices to the sea service, whether subjects of Her Majesty or not, who, by reason of having been discharged or left behind abroad, or shipwrecked from any British ship or any of Her Maj sty's ships, are in distress in any place abroad : and (b) seamen and apprentices to the sea service, being subjects of Her Majesty, who have been engaged by any person acting either as principal or agent to serve in a ship belonging to the Government or to a subject or citizen of a foreign country, and are in distress in any place abroad—shall be maintained by governors of British possessions, British consular officers, and other officers of Her Majesty in foreign countries, until a passage home can be procured. If there are no such officers, a British merchant may act.'

6. Another clause of the Consolidation Act refers to a native of any country in Asia, Africa, or of any of the islands in the South Sea or Pacific Ocean, or of any other country not having any consul in the United Kingdom, who is brought to the United Kingdom in any ship, British or foreign, as a seaman. If left in the United Kingdom he becomes chargeable, or commits any act that makes him liable as an ' idle and disorderly ' person, or any other act of vagrancy, the master or owner of the ship, or the consignee, if the

Seamen: natives of Asia, Africa, etc.

vessel be foreign, 'shall incur a penalty not exceeding thirty pounds, unless he can show that the person so left as aforesaid quitted the ship without the consent of the master, or that due means have been afforded by such master, owner or consignee, or one of them, to such person of returning to his native country or the country in which he was shipped; and the court inflicting such penalty may order the whole or any part of such penalty to be applied towards the relief or sending home of such person.'

Lascars and East Indians. 7. In the case of Lascars or other natives of the territories under the Government of the Council of India, who are found destitute in the United Kingdom, and relieved by Poor Law Guardians, notice may be sent to the Secretary of that Council, stating the name of the person, the presidency or district of which he professes to be a native, the ship in which he came, and the port and time of his arrival. The moneys expended in relief will then be repaid.

XXVII.—Shoeblacks, Commissionaires, and Messengers.

To test the energy of a boy it is sometimes useful to get him work as a shoeblack. The names and addresses of shoeblack brigades are given in the Register. The police give them licenses and appoint the places at which they are to stand. For molesting an authorised shoeblack, commissionaire, or messenger, or fraudulently pretending to be one, there is a penalty of 40s.[1] Particulars regarding the Corps of Commissionaires will be found in the Register.

XXVIII.—The Unemployed.

Causes of want of employment. Want of employment is occasioned by fluctuations in trade, or by the periodic nature of certain occupations, or by illness, misfortune, or some exceptional incapacity; intemperance and indolence are also the cause of much that goes by the name of want of work. Trade-unions are the mode by which the workman protects himself against the probable contingencies of his business; and in the case of riverside workers and others who lack any trade organisation, periodic charity can be no sufficient or proper substitute (see *ante*, p. v.). It is on this class that wholesale charity and out-relief act most cruelly. They know that, if unprovided for, some sort of miserable pittance is forthcoming, and this is enough to make them careless of providing for themselves. Other trades, *e.g.* that of painters, are also in their nature periodic, and families are frequently found to live with comparative extravagance during the high-wages season of summer, and to be dependent on credit, the help of neighbours, and charity

---

[1] Metropolitan Streets Act 1867 (30 & 31 Vict., c. 36), ss. 19 and 20.

in the winter. In these cases, charitable help, when there is a definite prospect of work, may be given conditionally on the parents putting by or joining a club, and personal influence should be forthcoming to enforce the obligation. Sickness will often add an additional plea for help; but, unless the applicant can be put into a new way of living, it would be better that the parish doctor should attend. The recklessness of one class of the poor as to whether they keep in work (caused, it must be remembered, in great measure by the conditions under which they are employed) is amazing. The vagrant who asks for employment will, as a rule, refuse it or leave it, if he is set to 'a job'; and there is in the Metropolis a host of enfeebled and incapable persons who often lack employment. They are the first to be discharged if work is slack, and their incompetence is an effective bar to their retaining work. Charity cannot usually assist in these instances. It is obvious that any attempt to do so, on a large scale, would depress wages, and would attract the labourers from their own trade organisations, or impede the formation of these organisations. Except perhaps in emergencies, charity should avoid interference with the supply of unskilled labour. Nor should it undertake the duties of an employer. As a test, a wood-yard has been found useful. But test work, provided under the Outdoor Relief Regulation Order by the Guardians, with proper classification, should, in co-operation with charity, serve this purpose better.

With regard to women's work we quote only a few sentences from a paper furnished in 1889 by Miss C. E. Collet, now one of the Labour Correspondents of the Board of Trade, to Mr. Charles Booth's 'Life and Labour: East London.' The sentences refer only to women's labour in and out of factories in East London, but the moral they suggest has a wider application. Miss Collet writes:—

The limits of charitable help in cases of want of employment.

Women's wages and work.

'On the whole, work in the factories is regular. More single women would be employed if work were not done at home, and domestic competition prevents wages from being so high as they would otherwise be. But it is obvious that any employer who uses machinery must be anxious to utilise his machinery and rooms to the utmost; and, on the whole, the irregularity in the employment of factory girls is due to the state of the trade, and not to any carelessness on the part of the employer, who would always like to give full work throughout the year if he could. The system of employing out-door hands makes it unnecessary to increase unduly the number of indoor hands in very busy times, and when trade returns to its normal condition the home workers are left unemployed, but the factory girls earn about the same as before.' Then after referring to the irregular hands employed in the confectionery and match trades, which are conducted wholly in factories ('the regular hands are a class apart, both socially and industrially'), Miss Collet puts the problem thus:—

'Which alternative should the employer choose? Should he divide the work among them all, or should he in slack times dismiss hands?

'This problem in some form or other must be faced by employers in every trade. Is half a loaf better than no bread? During a temporary scarcity it is. In the factory the expense of machinery and buildings tends to prevent the

employer from taking on more hands than are required in full work ; and in slack
times it seems best to divide work among them all. But, unless the girls have
saved in their best times, they naturally complain so much at their smaller earnings, that it sometimes pays the employer better to dismiss the inferior hands,
and to give the rest an opportunity of earning their usual amount. And the girls
never do save. If their standard of living included saving for slack times, they
could force wages up to that point in the season. But so long as they only wish
they could save, and always spend all their money, so long will full wages merely
correspond to necessary wages ; *i.e.* they will only be enough for present wants.

'The same question—whether half a loaf is better than no bread—presents
itself to the employer in another form. Granted that three girls at 10s. a week
are worth the same as four girls at 7s. 6d. a week, is it not better to give
employment to the four than the three? If the employer decides that he will
employ no one who is not worth 9s. a week, he really divides the work among a
smaller number of efficient girls. It may be true that no girl by herself can live
respectably on less than 9s. a week ; but it is also true that there are many girls
who would not be worth employing at that rate. In other words, there are girls
who, as things are, are not worth decent maintenance wages. The employer who
only employs girls who are worth this may preserve the even tenor of his way,
and congratulate himself that he at least is free from the guilt of employing
hands at starvation wages. But what about the large numbers who are thus
left unemployed? This is the question asked by a large number of manufacturers,
and their answer to those who demand that a minimum wage should be fixed is
that in that case they will have to dismiss many of their hands. What would be
done with the great mass of unemployed left to starve? I do not attempt to
answer this question. But two facts should be noticed. Fix a minimum rate of
wages, and an incentive is given to those whose working power has hitherto been
below par through indolence or lowness of standard, to raise themselves to the
required level. Those who are left are the physically or mentally incapable, or
the idle. Secondly, if these are left as wholly unemployed, they can be dealt
with much more easily than the half-paid or partly unemployed, who drag down
the population to their level. They are not left to starve. The parish rates and
charitable contributions, which at present are spent in doing harm to the many,
and in lowering wages, could be wholly devoted to the improvement of the
condition of the few, either in pleasure-houses or in workhouses, according to
the circumstances of the case. The inefficient are always irregularly employed.
Irregular employment causes irregular demand, and irregular demand causes
irregularity of employment. Each force acts with increased momentum.'

Provision of
employment
by charity.
It may be suggested that the evil should be repaired by giving
work at a fancy or fair rate of wages ; or by co-operation, by which
the profits of middlemen or 'sweaters' would be added to the wages
of the workwomen ; or by combination, and striking or negotiating
for higher wages. Suppose that the first suggestion be adopted,
and that, in order to carry it out, a benevolent despot, otherwise
called Charity, supply the material below cost price or free of
expense. Then the manufactured article may be sold just below
the market rate, and the workwoman may have a larger wage than
she could otherwise earn, made up in part of the price of her labour
and in part of the price of the material that the benevolent despot
has supplied ; but injury will be done to all women working at a
less advantage, that is, unassisted by Charity. Or the manufactured
article may be sold at the ordinary market rate. Then in the same
way the workwoman will have a larger wage, made up of the price
of her labour *plus* the gift—the price of the material that has been
supplied gratuitously. This may benefit a few cases, but the help

is in the nature of an allowance, regulated according to the amount of work produced. Given to the indigent, or to those who are rather poor than distressed, instead of to those whom it is desired to assist out of misfortune, it has the tendency of out-relief or periodic charity in keeping down wages. Given for a time as an exception, and on a definite plan, with other help to the distressed, it may be a useful means of assistance. In some pension cases also (see p. clxxv.) it may be useful. Yet, what charity gives to feeble hands it takes from strong hands. The demand it thus supplies would have been supplied in the way of business by others. The amount of work available in different occupations is to a great extent a fixed quantity. In women's work so great is the competition, and, for many reasons, so low is the scale of payment, that charitable interference in regard to it should be jealously watched. The poor often ask to be assisted by sewing machines and mangles. But unless they can make new custom, so assisted, they merely deprive others of their living; and charity, instead of helping, only takes half or a part of one poor man's loaf to give it to another.

By co-operation then, or by combination, rather than by charity, the conditions of labour are to be improved. In general, charity in these matters will but do mischief.[1]

In those cases in which the want of employment is due to misfortune, and properly remediable by charity, work may be found by careful advertising in suitable papers, and by private influence. Sometimes by the migration of families of children, and often by placing girls in service, by obtaining charing for women, etc., it is comparatively easy to help the unemployed. As a rule, particularly when the applicant is of any special trade, he is better qualified to find work for himself than the almoner for him. Applicants for employment frequently say that 'they don't want charity': yet their lack of employment is often due to distress or to some special circumstance which must be dealt with; and then, the cause of distress removed, employment is forthcoming, not because employment is given, but because the applicant becomes an efficient workman. The following instances are illustrative cases in which charity, chiefly by indirect methods, enables those who are in distress from want of work to regain their position and their employment.

How charity should help in cases of want of employment.

C. N.,'30, married, with two children; carman for six years for one firm; out of work several months. 'A steady man; clever at his work; left owing to reduction of staff; wages 30s. a week.' Belonged to the Hearts of Oak. The Committee made an allowance of 10s. a week for eleven weeks. Then, as there

[1] On the proposals for the establishment of Municipal Workshops, Labour Colonies, etc., we have not touched here. Those who are interested in these subjects can obtain various papers in regard to them from the London Charity Organisation Society.

was still no prospect of work, offered to assist C. N. to emigrate, and made a further two weeks' allowance whilst he was considering the matter. Eventually he said that he would like to go, but that his wife refused. Visited in October, about nine months after the date of application, the report is that he was in casual work during the summer, and now has got a regular place, though at lower wages.

J. E., 42, married; five children are at work. In a club for twenty years; worked fifteen years, on and off, for a firm of signal lamp makers, who spoke well of him. Both he and his wife, admittedly, had been given to drink at one time; but there was reason to suppose that they had given it up; the home was very bare and poor. The employers promised him work directly they had it to give, and the Committee made an allowance from February to the end of May. Visited in October, the report is that J. E. has fairly regular work from his firm, and there are no signs of drink.

M., 26, glass-blower; worked for many years for one firm, but their trade was reported very slack and, apparently, without prospect of improvement. His employer reported him steady and industrious, but did not hold out much prospect of increased employment, there being at that moment a great number of glass-blowers out of work. Eventually, after some hesitation, the Committee made an allowance for two months. Then, as the circumstances did not improve, they offered emigration. Visited in October, M. is still working half-time for the same firm, and the report is that his rent is paid up and that he is in a much better position than he was last year.

'The above cases,' writes a District Committee of the Charity Organisation Society, 'show that charitable aid can under certain conditions assist distress which is due to want of employment; that it can help to tide over periods of slackness for men who have been in regular employment, and who have prospects of work within a reasonable time; or that it can, in the last resort, if they can get no further work in this country, help them to go to a better labour market. The Committee believe that distress from want of employment should be dealt with case by case. They can give no other answer to the "unemployed problem," except that if dealt with in this way they believe that it will be least likely to become unmanageable. They may say, for their own part, that they are always ready to entertain the cases of careful, industrious men who are exceptionally out of work; whilst they believe that the idle, the improvident, and the chronically unemployed can only be dealt with by the Poor Law.'

The following are two other cases of success, and one of failure :—

L——. First mate in the merchant service. He had failed in his examination for the Board of Trade certificate, and the firm of shipowners who employed him had refused to employ him again until he obtained a master's certificate. He was nine months out of work, and spent all his money on 'coaching' and in keeping his wife and family. In January the family were starving. They had sold their 'home' and had exhausted their friends' help, and were on the verge of despair. He applied to one of the relief committees, who gave him 7s. 6d. a week for two weeks. He then found his way to the Charity Organisation Society. The Committee decided to spare no expense in setting him on his legs again. They made him an allowance of 13s. 9d. a week and paid his fee of £2. 2s. for the examination. He failed once, twice, but was successful in his third and last chance. With the Board of Trade certificate he soon got a ship, and is now earning £9. 9s. a month, and repaying part of the money spent on him. His family is slowly recovering from the straits to which they were reduced, and he is full of thankfulness to those who inspired him with hope when all seemed over.

Mark R—— was once a sailor, but had to leave the navy owing to defective eye-sight. He has no pension. For many years he supported his family (wife and four children) by different kinds of rough labour. His eye-sight has been gradually growing worse for a long time, until now he is unable to get work anywhere. He was sent to us by the vicar of the parish, who had known him for many years. His wife is a monthly nurse, and has not been fortunate in getting employment, owing to the poverty of the district in which she has been living. She has now moved to a district where she is better known, and is more likely to earn money. Meanwhile her husband went into Moorfields Eye Hospital. It was found that one eye must be removed in order to save the other. After the operation we sent him to a convalescent home for three weeks. He came back and tried to get work, but failed. The worry and anxiety made his eye bad again, and we sent him to the country for another change. We have now succeeded in getting him work for winter months suitable to his infirmity.

G——, a docker, with children. He had lost his wife earlier in the year, and the home was being kept together by the eldest child, a girl of 14, who worked in a laundry. He was given three weeks' relief by the Rectors' Relief Committee, and referred to the Charity Organisation Society for further help. Enquiry proved that he was a drunken, lazy fellow, and that since his wife's death everything had gone to rack and ruin. The children were neglected, and picked up just enough to keep themselves alive—by free meals three times a week from a working men's club, and by what they could otherwise get. Their elder sister did her best for them. The Committee asked a lady to visit regularly and see what could be done. The children's relations were communicated with, and the relieving officer was informed of their condition. The best was done to get some of the children away from home into better surroundings, but eventually the man got work, and refused to co-operate with the Committee in their plans for helping him with his children. The cause of distress was temporarily removed, but the family was not permanently helped. It is impossible to help a man against his will.

In the Register will be found particulars in regard to some leading Trade Societies; also a list of employment agencies and servants' registries.

XXIX.—Emigration.

Emigration is a frequently-proposed remedy for helping the unemployed poor. A reference to the Register will show the cost of passages, the outfit required, etc. Like other modes of charitable aid, it is injurious if applied wholesale. If, as Mr. Fawcett has pointed out, the population continues to increase at the same rate, there will not be, except for a short time, fewer hands and more work in the Old Country. Without self-help and a higher standard of living, such assistance, coming from without, will be of very partial advantage. Generally speaking, the expense of emigration is so small that those who are likely to become good emigrants are those who can save enough to emigrate; the cost is a fair test of fitness. But, as in other instances, charity is in no way fettered by the application itself. If emigration is a good remedy in a particular case, and can be applied without removing natural obligations, charity may well use it, as in other instances it would obtain admission to a home. The most successful emigration often consists in sending to relations already settled in a colony, men and women or families likely to do well with their help. It might almost be said that emigration should in these times be restricted to such cases. No emigration case should be settled without the expert advice of persons who know the colonies intimately. Care should be taken to send persons to some suitable agent, through a trustworthy society, unless they go to relations; and arrangements should be made to meet necessary expenses on

Limits of emigration as a means of assistance.

f

landing and to give the new arrivals a fair start. Many wish and ask to be assisted to emigrate, who, even if generally suitable as emigrants, can be equally well aided in other ways. Sometimes, when a medical opinion is given to the effect that a breadwinner, out of health in England, would be strong and able to support himself in a Colony, *e.g.* at the Cape, he and his family have been sent out.

The following is an account of a case of family emigration and the emigration of relations to relations:—

'This case is rather the migration of a clan than of a family. In 1888 a single man, E. W——, a labourer, who was doing badly in Hackney Wick, emigrated to Manitoba, and reported so well of the country that in 1889 his parents followed him. Every year since then other members of the family have joined him; the sons have sent home for their sweethearts; now the tribe together amounts to about twenty-five, and they are at present saving to help out collateral branches of the clan. I dropped in unexpectedly at the house of the father one evening when all the family were assembled in honour of a birthday, and I never saw a more prosperous, a better dressed, or a happier collection of working men and women in my life. Yet in England, as these people told me, they existed with the fear of the workhouse perpetually before their eyes. Now some have constant work in manufactories, others in railway shops, and their future and that of the rapidly increasing number of grandchildren may be considered perfectly assured. In this case the Emigration Sub-Committee, the Hackney Committee, and the East-End Fund co-operated.'[1]

Powers of the Guardians in regard to emigration.

The Guardians, or rather the Local Government Board if set in motion by them, have large powers in regard to emigration. If a majority of owners and ratepayers assembled at a duly convened meeting so direct, they may, with the approval of the Local Government Board, pay from a fund specially raised for the purpose, the expenses of poor persons settled in their Union and willing to emigrate. This fund, it is stipulated, must not exceed half the average annual rate for the three preceding years, and is repayable in five years.[2]

By order of the Poor Law Board and in conformity with their regulations the Guardians may,[3] at the expense of the common fund of the Union, procure, or assist in procuring the emigration of any poor person who is irremovable by reason of a residence of one year.[4]

Further, the Guardians may,[5] with the order and subject to the rules of the Local Government Board, expend, without being authorised to do so by any previous meeting of owners and ratepayers, any sum not exceeding £10 'in and about' the emigration of any poor person settled in the Union, so long as the total moneys so expended do not exceed one half the average poor rate during the last three years.

[1] Report of the Council of the Charity Organisation Society, 1890–91.
[2] 4 & 5 Will. IV., c. 76, s. 62.   [3] 11 & 12 Vict., c. 110, s. 5.
[4] 9 & 10 Vict., c. 66, s. 1, as modified by 24 & 25 Vict., c. 55, s. 1, and 28 & 29 Vict., c. 79, s. 8.
[5] 12 & 13 Vict., c 103, s. 20.

The Guardians can thus, if there is a crisis requiring such remedies, provide for the emigration of a large number of persons; they can also assist individual cases, even though they are not at the time paupers. The confirmation of the Local Government Board is necessary, and therefore the decision rests in their hands. Owing to representations from the Government of the United States, the Local Government Board are 'precluded, except in very special cases, from sanctioning emigration to that country at the cost of the poor rate.'[1] Apart from orphan or deserted children, in 1892 only 59 persons were assisted to emigrate through Boards of Guardians, at a cost of £209. 10s.

Under the Local Government Act 1888, the County Councils may from time to time, with the consent of the Local Government Board, borrow for, amongst other purposes, 'making advances (which they are hereby authorised to make) to any persons or bodies of persons, corporate or unincorporate, in aid of the emigration or colonisation of inhabitants of the county, with a guarantee for the repayment of such advances from any local authority in the county or the Government of any colony.'[2] This clause gives to a new and more widely representative body the option of raising a fund for emigration. But it does not interfere with the powers already possessed by the Guardians. Further, the fund is to be raised under two very exact restrictions. Only advances are made by it, and these are repayable on guarantee, either by the Colony or by the local authority; and the only local authority that would appear to be competent to give a guarantee for repayment is the Board of Guardians. But if the Board of Guardians deal with these emigration cases, the objections now taken to 'pauper' emigration hold good. On the other hand, if the Colony gives the guarantee, it has indirectly a complete check on the amount of money expended, and the conditions imposed, in sending emigrants to it. *Power of County Councils in regard to emigration.*

To the enactments by which the machinery of the Poor Law can be utilised for purposes of emigration, the not unreasonable objection, just referred to, is taken, that the Colonies are unwilling to admit emigrants who bear the reproach of being 'pauper' emigrants. But, even if this be granted, it is almost certain that no other State-aided system would serve the purpose better. Highly organised attempts at emigration in large bodies have seldom met with success; and when philanthropists most desire emigration for others, people in general, if we may trust the returns, are rather less inclined to emigrate, for the rise in emigration is generally coincident with improving, the fall with declining, trade. On the whole, then, State-aided emigration or emigration organised on a large scale cannot be advocated. It is better to trust to individual enterprise. *State-aided emigration.*

[1] Glen's Archbold, p. 306. [2] Local Government Act 1888 (51 & 52 Vict., c. 41). s. 69.

In the case of orphan or deserted children who are under the age of 16 and chargeable to the Union, and who have no place of settlement, or whose place of settlement is unknown, the Guardians, with the consent of the Local Government Board, may procure or assist in procuring emigration.[1] The consent of the child must be given before justices in petty sessions, and a certificate of this consent has to be transmitted to the Local Government Board.

The Guardians may, subject to the sanction of the Local Government Board, send orphan and deserted pauper children to Canada, under the following conditions[2]:—

(1) That they obtain 'in each case an undertaking in writing from any person entrusted by them with the care of taking children to Canada, and of placing them in homes, that immediately after a child is placed out the Department of Agriculture at Ottawa shall be furnished with a report containing the name and age of the child, and the name and post office address of the person with whom the child is placed, and that a report containing similar information shall be furnished to the Guardians of the Union from which the child is taken.'

(2) That they send a copy of the report to the Local Government Board.

(3) That they give notice to the person proposed to be entrusted by them with the emigration of a child, whether the child is Protestant or Roman Catholic, and 'he shall give an undertaking if the child is a Protestant that he shall be placed with a family of the Protestant faith, or if the child is a Roman Catholic, that he shall be placed in a Roman Catholic home.'

(4) That 'a child before being sent to Canada shall have been under previous instruction at least six months, in a workhouse, separate, or district school, or at a public elementary school at the cost of the Guardians, or in a school certified by the Local Government Board.'

(5) That each child is examined by the medical officer, who has 'to report in writing as to its health, both of body and mind,' and to certify whether it is 'in all respects a suitable subject for emigration.'

(6) That the Guardians have such evidence as they deem satisfactory, that the person taking out the children has reasonable prospect of finding suitable homes for them in Canada.'

'The Board consider that as a general rule girls should not be sent out above the age of 10 years, and in no case, except under very special circumstances, above the age of 12 years.'

These regulations may suggest to charitable persons, desirous of sending children to Canada, the general conditions upon which

[1] 13 & 14 Vict., c. 101, s. 4.
[2] Memorandum of Local Government Board, April 1888.

they should insist, if they are to accomplish so difficult a task without any great risk of failure.

XXX.—MARRIED WOMEN.

I.—RIGHTS IN THEIR OWN PROPERTY.[1]
II.—REMEDIES AGAINST ILL-TREATMENT OR NEGLECT.
III.—GUARDIANSHIP OF THEIR CHILDREN.

I. *Property.*—The rights of married women with respect to their property are established by the Married Woman's Property Act 1882 (45 & 46 Vict., c. 75).

A married woman is capable of acquiring, holding, and disposing, by will or otherwise, of any real or personal property as her separate property in the same manner as if she were a *feme sole*, without the intervention of any trustee; and she may, in respect of and to the extent of her separate property, present and future, enter into any contract, and sue or be sued alone; and she may carry on a trade separate from her husband, and in that case be subject to the bankruptcy laws. All property, including wages and earnings, to which she may become entitled after January 1, 1883, become her separate property with the same rights. A woman married after that date is entitled to keep the whole of her property, present and future, as her separate property.

All deposits in savings or other banks, annuities, and other securities, standing in her name alone, belong to her till the contrary be shown; and she may receive dividends, and transfer without the concurrence of her husband; and where they stand in her name jointly with others, she may act as if she were a *feme sole*. If, however, she make any fraudulent investment of the husband's money in her own name, or to defraud his creditors, it will be invalid.

She may effect a policy of insurance on her own life, or her husband's, for her separate use, and a husband or wife who insures his or her life expressly for the benefit of the other, or of his or her children, with or without a trustee, shall create a trust in favour of the objects named in the policy; but if done to defraud creditors, they shall be entitled to receive the amount of premiums so wrongfully paid.

Every married woman has the same remedies, civil and criminal, for the protection of her property as if she were a *feme sole*, but she cannot take criminal proceedings against her husband whilst they are living together, nor for any act done by him whilst they were living together, unless with regard to property taken by him when leaving or deserting her, and she is herself liable to criminal

[1] The substance of this section was furnished for a previous edition by a member of the Society.

proceedings in respect of any act done to his property which if done by him to her property would make him criminally liable.

A woman after her marriage continues bound in respect of and to the extent of her separate property by all liabilities incurred before her marriage, and may be sued alone in respect of them. Her husband is only bound to satisfy her previous liabilities to the extent of any property he may have received from her.

A married woman who is an executrix or administratrix, or a trustee, either alone or with others, may sue and be sued, and transfer the property as if she were a *feme sole*.

The Act does not interfere with settlements made before or after marriage, nor render inoperative any restriction against anticipation, but no such restriction to be made by her in respect of her own property shall be valid against debts contracted before marriage, and no settlement shall have any greater validity as against her creditors than would be given to a husband's settlement as against his creditors.

If her husband become chargeable to the parish, she is liable to support him out of her separate property, and she must in like manner maintain her children and grandchildren[1] in the same way as the husband is now liable to do, but without relieving him of his liability.

The Act does not extend to Scotland.

Married women, even before the Act, had, since August 9, 1870, been entitled as their own property to their wages and earnings in any employment, occupation, or trade carried on separately from their husbands, and to all investments of such wages and earnings.

II. *Person.*—A married woman whose husband ill-treats or neglects to maintain her has the following remedies :—

Husband and wife : Procedure in assault cases.

1. A summons, in case of personal violence, threatened or offered by her husband, to appear before a justice to show cause why he should not be bound over to keep the peace, and if necessary to find sureties. One justice can hear such a summons; but if it should come before two, they can if they see fit convert it into a charge of assault, and deal with it as such.

2. A summons under 24 & 25 Vict., cap. 100, sec. 42, with a view to his being imprisoned for not exceeding two months, or fined. This is the ordinary law as to common assault, but subject, as between husband and wife, to two important amplifications, viz. :—

(*a*) Contrary to the ordinary rule, they can give evidence against one another in such case.

(*b*) By section 43 of the Act, the period of imprisonment may be extended to six months, if in the opinion of the justices an assault (on a woman or child) is of such an 'aggravated' nature that it cannot be sufficiently punished under section 42.

---

[1] This point is doubtful. See *ante*, p. li.

If, on the hearing of such summons, the justices think that the case will be better met by requiring the defendant to be bound over to keep the peace or to find sureties, they can do so. Under section 43 they can both punish and bind over.

In proceeding under either 1 or 2, a warrant, instead of a summons, may be granted if there appear to be danger of immediate violence to the wife—a danger that is sometimes increased by the fact of a summons only being issued. A warrant is an order to the constable to arrest the offender and bring him before a justice.

3. *Protection Order.*—This gives no further protection to the wife than is already afforded by law, and is now unnecessary, but is sometimes still usefully shown to the police, although in the absence of such order she has, when living apart from her husband, the right to protect herself against invasion by him by calling in the aid of the police.[1]

4a. *Judicial Separation.*—By the Matrimonial Causes Act 1878 (41 & 42 Vict., cap. 19), section 4, justices *who have convicted the husband of an aggravated assault upon the wife* (2 *b*), and are satisfied that the *future safety of the wife is in peril*, may further make an order for a judicial separation, for the payment of a weekly sum by the husband, and for the custody by the wife of the children under ten years of age.

4b. *Separation Agreement.*—These have been valid ever since the Reformation, both at law and in equity, and it may be noted that, now that it is competent for husband and wife to contract with each other; a trustee is no longer required.

5. *Desertion.*—By the Married Women's (Maintenance in case of Desertion) Act 1886 (49 & 50 Vict., cap. 53), justices or a magistrate may make an order upon the summons of a wife deserted by her husband, who wilfully neglects to maintain her and her family, though able to do so wholly or in part, that the husband pay to the wife such weekly sum (not exceeding two pounds) as they may consider to be in accordance with his means, and with any means the wife may have for the support of her and her family. *Legal responsibilities of the husband.*

The above are the only remedies for which the wife can apply directly, but there are two others which she can obtain by making herself chargeable to the poor-rate. The Guardians of the Poor should then proceed against the husband, either

6. Under 31 & 32 Vict., cap. 122, sec. 33, for the cost of the relief given to the wife; or,

7. Under 5 Geo. IV., cap. 83, sec. 3, for neglecting to maintain

---

[1] *See* Lush's 'Husband and Wife,' p. 19. The practical effect of the judgment in the Jackson case (1891) is that if a wife leaves her husband on account of his ill-treatment, he has no legal power to compel her by force to return to him, although it must be borne in mind that if she leaves him without such cause as would have justified her in leaving him before that judgment, it will be at the risk of her right to be maintained by him.

his wife and family, though able to do so wholly or in part, for which he is liable to one month's hard labour, without option of fine ; for a second offence to three months; and for a third to twelve months.

In this case (7) the wife cannot give evidence (45 J.P. 687).

There seems to be some doubt whether and how far the Guardians have power to obtain permanent maintenance for a deserted wife from her husband, and some Boards of Guardians require the woman to accept indoor relief, that is, to enter the workhouse (which sometimes involves her breaking up a separate home), before they will set the law (6 and 7) in motion, but it is not necessary for them to oblige her to do so.

Uncondoned adultery by a wife is a defence to 5, 6, and 7.

If a husband or wife be absent for seven years without any information concerning him or her reaching the other party, and the latter marry, he or she cannot be convicted of bigamy ; but no length of such absence makes such a marriage valid, should the absent party prove to have been alive when it was contracted (45 J.P. 414).

III. *Children.*—By the Guardianship of Infants Act 1886 (49 & 50 Vict., cap. 27) :

1. On the death of the father of an infant the mother, if surviving, shall be the guardian, either alone or jointly with any guardian appointed by the father.

In the absence or a failure of the guardian appointed by the father, the Court may appoint a guardian to act jointly with the mother.

2. The mother of an infant may by deed or will appoint a guardian after the death of herself and the father ; if guardians are appointed by both parents, they shall act jointly.

The mother of an infant may by deed or will provisionally nominate a fit person to act as guardian after her death jointly with the father, and the Court may after her death confirm the appointment, if it be shown that the father is for any reason unfitted to be the sole guardian.

3. If the guardians are unable to agree upon a question affecting the welfare of the infant, any of them may apply to the Court for direction.

4. The Court may, upon the application of the mother of an infant, who may apply without a next friend, make an order regarding the custody of the infant and the right of access thereto of either parent, having regard to the welfare of the infant and to the conduct of the parents, and to the wishes as well of the mother as of the father.

5. The Court, in pronouncing a decree for judicial separation or for divorce, *nisi* or absolute, may declare the parent, by reason of

whose misconduct such decree is made, to be unfit to have the custody of the children of the marriage; and such parent shall not, upon the death of the other parent, be entitled as of right to the custody or guardianship of the children.

The Court includes the County Court of the district in which the respondent resides.

XXXI.—NON-PROVISION FOR WIDOWS AND CHILDREN.

Very many applicants for charitable relief belong to no club. Many are insured in collecting burial or industrial insurance societies, but few for a sum larger than that which is necessary to meet the actual expenses of funeral. On the other hand, the membership of friendly societies is on the increase; and collecting societies are doing a larger business in ordinary adult insurance among the poorer classes than was ever done before. But by degrees insurance for the payment of funeral expenses is being succeeded by insurance for some reasonable amount, such as £100, payable at death or after the lapse of a certain period, as an 'endowment.' Provision is thus made for widows, and, if the demand arises, it may be made in some more specific form for old age. Popular sentiment has been the trading basis of the collecting burial societies; it is now supplying them with as good a basis for ordinary insurance. The number of applicants that belong to clubs has often been reckoned. At the Greenwich Charity Organisation Committee, for instance, in 1884-5, out of 433 applicants, 270 belonged to no club, while of those who were entered as belonging to clubs, 43 were in industrial insurance societies, such as the Prudential or the Royal Liver; and 56 belonged to slate clubs. Often and often it is found also that the club money paid to a widow has been quickly spent, and she comes for assistance just as she is spending the last penny of a sum which, carefully used, might have enabled her to keep independent.

(marginal note: Frequent lack of provision for widows and children.)

To deal with these cases properly it is necessary to have some knowledge of the means at the disposal of the Guardians, and the requirements of the School Board. The means at the disposal of charity, such as orphanages and homes, will be found by reference to the Register.

XXXII.—POOR LAW PROVISION FOR CHILDREN: SCHOOLS.

The Poor Law schools are of two kinds: (1) District schools, *i.e.* schools provided under the Poor Law Amendment Act of 1844 and subsequent Acts, in two or more Unions, which are for this purpose combined in school districts; and (2) Separate workhouse schools, provided for a single Union. Those in the Metropolis are, with one exception, built in the suburbs. The district schools are under the management of a separate Board, elected by the Guardians in the school district. The separate schools are under

(marginal note: District and separate schools.)

the management of the Schools Committee of the Board of Guardians of the Unions to which they belong.

By the Metropolitan Poor Act 1867, the Local Government Board was empowered to combine metropolitan Parishes and Unions into school districts. For reference sake they may be mentioned here. The school available in each Union is also set down in the local lists.

PARISHES AND UNIONS COMBINED IN DISTRICT SCHOOLS.

Parish or Union.	Name of School District.	Situation of School.
1. City and St. Saviour's	Central London	Hanwell.
2. Poplar and Whitechapel	Forest Gate	Stratford, E.
3. Kensington and Chelsea	Kensington and Chelsea	Banstead.[1]
4. Lewisham and Wandsworth, and Clapham	North Surrey	Anerley.
5. Camberwell, Greenwich, St. Olave's, Stepney, Woolwich	South Metropolitan	Sutton and Witham, Essex.[2]
6. Fulham, Paddington, St. George's	West London	Ashford, Middlesex.

SEPARATE SCHOOLS.

The following Unions have these schools:—

Parish or Union.	Situation of School.
St. George-in-the-East	Plashet.
Islington (a workhouse school in a detached building)	Holloway.
Lambeth	Norwood.
Bethnal Green	Leytonstone.
St. Pancras	Leavesden.
Holborn	Mitcham.
Marylebone	Southall.
Mile End Old Town (a workhouse school in a detached building)	Mile End.
Strand	Edmonton.
Westminster	Tooting.
Hackney	Brentwood.
Shoreditch	Hornchurch.

St. Giles' send the children to the Strand Union School at Edmonton; Hampstead to the Edmonton Union and Westminster Union separate schools.

Outsiders seldom realise how elaborate and carefully devised are the new 'workhouse' schools. The Kensington and Chelsea District School is on the cottage home system, which is now frequently adopted. Thus for the parish of Shoreditch cottage homes have been erected at Hornchurch, Essex. They are described as eleven in number, each with accommodation for a foster mother and 30 children, and ' built in the detached villa style on either side of a broad main street.' In the village there are workshops, a bakehouse, swimming bath, stores, chapel, school-room, band-room, infirmary, infectious-disease hospital, &c. The buildings occupy about 14 acres, and the remaining land, about 60 acres, is utilised as a sewage farm. For the erection of these schools an expenditure of £51,000 was sanctioned by the Local Government Board in 1887.

[1] Probationary School at Hammersmith.

[2] This is a branch school for orphans and deserted children between the ages of 7 and 12. The managers of the same school district hire a school at Sutton for infants.

In connection with Unions in the country are schools consisting of still smaller and more homelike cottage houses. To such large and well-appointed schools the poor have often but little compunction in sending their children.

The Poor Law schools are 'public elementary schools under the Elementary Education Act of 1876,' but they are under periodic inspection by School inspectors appointed by the Local Government Board. Certificates are given to the teachers according to their proficiency. To provide a bonus on the appointment of competent teachers, the salaries of teachers are supplemented by Parliamentary grants according to the 'grade' of their certificate, and the number of children they teach. Industrial instructors are also appointed. The schools are very large. In the Central London District School (City and St. Saviour's), there was during the half-year ended at Lady Day, 1892, an average daily attendance of 818 children. At the South Metropolitan District School the return of children was 2,304. The total number of children at the 16 metropolitan district and separate schools, including 491 boys in the 'Exmouth,' the training ship of the Metropolitan Asylum District, was 11,527.

With regard to discipline, a boy under the age of 14 may be flogged, but two hours must have elapsed from the commission of the offence: an older boy may be caned. Children under 12 may not be confined in a dark room, or during the night; and all cases of punishment in a workhouse or pauper school have to be reported to the Guardians.

If a child is 'refractory,' or the child of parents either of whom has been convicted of a crime or offence punishable with penal servitude or imprisonment, and whom it is desirable to remove, two justices may, on the representation of a Board of Guardians, send him to a certified industrial school [1] (see p. cxxi.). During the enquiry or pending removal he may, by the order of the justices, be kept in the workhouse.

Besides their own schools, the Guardians have the following means of educating children [2] :—

(1) If in any Union there is room in the 'workhouse or building having adequate provision for the reception, maintenance, and education of poor children,' the Guardians can contract with other Unions for the reception of children under the age of 16, who are orphans

Other provisions by which Guardians may help children.

---

[1] 29 & 30 Vict., c. 118, s. 17.

[2] In many Unions children are sent for their education to the local public elementary schools. In the Metropolis, whenever any child supposed to have strayed has been received into a workhouse, the Master has to place a notice on the workhouse-gate, and send a notice to each of the three nearest police-stations. If within twenty-four hours no claim or inquiry is made, he has to send a copy to the Clerk of the Board of Guardians, 36 copies to the Commissioners of the Metropolitan Police, and 12 to the Commissioner of the City Police.

or deserted by their parents, or whose parents or surviving parent consent.[1]

Sending children to voluntary schools.

(2) They may send a child, if orphan or deserted by his or her parents or surviving parent (or one whose parents or surviving parent shall consent thereto),[2] till the age of 14, to any certified school, supported wholly or in part by voluntary subscriptions, provided that the cost does not exceed what would have been the cost in the workhouse, during the period at which the child is at the school. These schools are open to inspection by the Poor Law inspectors or by members of the Board of Guardians which has sent a child.

This provision includes any institution for the instruction of the blind, deaf, dumb, lame, deformed, or idiotic, but not a certified reformatory school.[3] Children cannot be sent to a school conducted on the principles of a religious denomination to which they do not belong.

The consent of the parents is required in the case of illegitimate as well as legitimate children; for the former, the consent of the mother, if she has the care of the child, is sufficient. The Local Government Board has discretion in the case of deserted or orphan children as to the choice of the school to which, owing to religious grounds, the child should be sent, when no next-of-kin, step-parent, or god-parent can be found.[4]

XXXIII.—POOR LAW PROVISION FOR CHILDREN : TRAINING SHIPS.

Training ships.

(3) Training ships.—The Guardians of any Union, and the managers of any school or asylum district in the Metropolis may, with the consent of the Local Government Board, provide one or more ships to be used for training boys for the sea service.[5] Such a ship is considered a school or asylum. The parent's consent (if surviving) has to be obtained, and a certificate from the Union medical officer that the boy is free from disease, and fit for training for the sea service. On admission to the ship he is placed in a probationary ward and medically examined. If eventually found unfit, or if there be proof of gross misconduct, he is discharged to the district or separate school or workhouse. The training-ship under the Metropolitan Asylums Board is the 'Exmouth.' In the half-year ended Lady-day 1892 the average daily number of boys in training there was 491.

---

[1] 14 & 15 Vict., c. 105, s. 6.

[2] 25 & 26 Vict., c. 43, ss. 1, 2, 4, 6. As to amount payable, the Local Government Board sanctions six shillings as the weekly sum to be paid for each child. *Cf.* Glen's Archbold, p. 291.

[3] *Ibid.*, s. 10. In regard to the Elementary Education (Blind and Deaf) Children Act 1893, and its bearing on the work of Guardians in dealing with blind and deaf and dumb children, *see* p. cxxix.

[4] 31 & 32 Vict., c. 122, s. 23.

[5] 32 & 33 Vict., c. 63, s. 11, and Local Government Board Order, August 24, 1876.

XXXIV.—POOR LAW PROVISION FOR CHILDREN: BOARDING-OUT.

(4) Another means at the disposal of the Guardians for pro- *Boarding-out: condi-*
viding for orphan or deserted children, is boarding-out. It is *tions under*
regulated in England by the Poor Law Order of May 28, 1889. *which it is permitted.*
Formerly the Guardians could only board-out children within
their Unions; since the Boarding-out Orders have been issued they
have been able to board them beyond the limits of the Union—a
necessary provision if the Unions in large towns were to adopt the
system. The children are placed in cottagers' houses, under the
care of foster-parents, and under the supervision of a Boarding-out
Committee. The following are the principal requirements:—

A Boarding-out Committee is formed of three or more members:
each member has to sign an undertaking truly and faithfully to
observe all regulations prescribed in the Order, and is disqualified if
he derive any pecuniary or personal profit from the boarding-out of
any child. Children can be withdrawn by the Guardians at a
week's notice. The Committee is responsible for finding and superintending the homes at which the children are boarded.

The children who may be boarded-out must be between the
ages of two and ten, except in the case of a child above the age of
ten years placed in the same home with a brother or sister under
that age, and they must be either orphans or deserted. The term
'orphan child' in the Boarding-out Order means 'a child both of
whose parents are dead, or one of whose parents is dead, the other
being under sentence of penal servitude, or suffering permanently
from mental disease, or being permanently bedridden or disabled
and an inmate of a workhouse, or being out of England.' The term
'deserted child' means 'a child deserted by both parents, or
deserted by one parent, the other being dead, etc., as above; or a
child one of whose parents is under penal servitude,' etc. A certificate
of health has, prior to its being boarded-out, to be sent by the medical
officer of the Union to the Boarding-out Committee. Except in the
case of brothers and sisters, not more than two children can be
boarded in the same house, and never more than four. They
cannot be placed with foster-parents of different religious per-
suasions, and the foster-parents have to undertake 'to bring
them up as their own children,' to provide proper food, &c.,
to see that the child goes to school and to church or chapel, and
to report any sickness to the Guardians and the Boarding-out
Committee. The sum payable is not more than 4s. a week exclusive
of clothing, school pence, and medical fees. There must be a school
within a mile and a half from the home, and the residence of a member of the Committee must be within five miles. The child must be
visited and reported on at least once in every six weeks by a
member of the Committee, the report being sent not less often than
quarterly to the Guardians. If no report is received for four consecu-

tive months, the Guardians may provide for the home being visited once in every six weeks by their own officer, or withdraw the child.

Some further details showing the care which, as all admit, has to be taken in boarding-out children are given by the Local Government Board in their circular. They may be suggestive to persons desirous of paying for the boarding-out of children from charitable funds. Children, except in special cases, are not to be placed with relations, or those who are in receipt of Poor Law relief, or who have been in receipt of it during the past twelve months, or where the father has night work. Preference is to be given to the parents who have outdoor and not sedentary occupations. Decent accommodation and proper separation of the sexes must be provided. Children over seven are not allowed to sleep in the same room with married couples. No child is to be boarded in a house where there is an adult lodger. Not more than two children (or unless they be brothers and sisters, not more than four in number) may be boarded-out at one home at one time. Nor may a child be boarded-out where there are five other children in the family. If after two warnings to the foster-parents the schoolmaster's quarterly report is unfavourable, the child is to be withdrawn. Good ordinary clothing is to be provided at not more than 10s. a quarter. Children should not be sent to homes in places having a population of more than 15,000 persons.

Pro and con. regarding boarding-out.

The boarding-out system is strongly advocated and as strongly opposed. Its advocates urge that it gives the child a quasi-natural position as the member of a family, and that it merges the child in the population ; as he grows up he learns a trade and obtains work as others do in that rank of life. If the means of instruction are less complete than in a district school, there is more of education in its larger sense. A knowledge of life and a friendship with others is obtained, which is not to be had in a district school. And, especially with girls, is it necessary to substitute for the institutional life of a large school the family life. This gives a knowledge of those household matters, in regard to which girls from large schools often show a marked incapacity, and influences the character most beneficially. Lastly, the system has been very successful in Scotland. The opponents point to the favourable results of the district schools, and the greater educational resources of a large institution. Strict supervision is difficult. The efficiency of the Local Boarding-out Committee is very variable, and the system is injurious to district schools by withdrawing the orphan children, the most permanent element. The payment of 4s. a week, with the cost of school fees, clothing, and medical attendance, places the child of a pauper in a better position than the child of the labourer, the foster-parent, who seldom has 4s. to spend on one child. This will lead him to compare the lot of his own children unfavourably with that of the children, and often the illegitimate children, of improvident pauper parents. So he will be taught a lesson in unthrift. It will encourage illegitimacy also, it is said ; it is more attractive to the poor than institutions, and the advantages of family life will be purchased at too great a sacrifice in other ways.

The practice of boarding-out children on payment from charitable sources is not infrequent in dealing with the cases of widows who have to go into service, etc. A list of Boarding-out Committees will be found in the Register. The number of children boarded outside the Union under the Order of May, 1889, was, on January 1, 1892, 1,738. There is an inspector (Miss Mason) for the purpose of visiting children boarded-out in different parts of the country.

An instance of assisting a widow by a combination of boarding-out and admission to homes is given in the following case :—

A poor widow was very ill, and had been ordered by the doctor to go into the *Illustrative case.* hospital, where a lengthened course of treatment would be necessary. She did not know how to manage it, as her eldest boy was only fifteen, and was out all day, and the other children were too young to be left alone. The clergyman in whose parish the woman lived sent the case on to the Committee, not having funds to deal with it adequately. She was very much respected by all who knew her, and her life depended on going into the hospital at once. Great efforts were made by the Committee, and kind assistance was given by a clergyman. Two children were placed in orphanages. The eldest girl was boarded-out, and a place subsequently found for her. The baby was boarded-out with a woman who bestowed on it all the care and attention that could be desired, under the supervision of the clergyman's wife. The mother was most grateful for what had been done. She has since come out of the hospital fairly restored in health, and is prospering. Though still not strong, she has a light place, and is contributing 2s. 6d. a week towards the support of her baby.

XXXV.—POOR LAW PROVISION FOR CHILDREN : APPRENTICESHIP.[1]

(5) Apprenticeship or sending out to service is another resource *Condition* open to Guardians. The Guardians can apprentice any poor child *of apprenticeship by* not under nine years old, who can (unless deaf and dumb) read and *the Guardians.* write his own name.[2] It is not necessary that either child or parent should be actually in receipt of relief as paupers at the time. Apprenticeship is to be considered a species of 'relief,' and should not, therefore, except with the sanction of the Local Government Board, be provided, for instance, in the case of the child of an able-bodied man, unless the latter be in receipt of relief in the house or otherwise according to the Outdoor Relief Prohibitory or Regulation Orders.

If the child is in the workhouse and under the age of 14, the medical officer has to give a certificate of his bodily fitness for the proposed trade, and the master of the workhouse has to vouch for his

[1] It may be well to mention that, under the Stamp Act of 1870, public charities are exempted from the payment of indenture fees in putting out apprentices.
[2] Consolidated Order, art. 52. Cf. Macmorran: Poor Law General Orders, p. 71.

general capacity. If the child is not in the workhouse, the relieving officer has to inquire and report on the circumstances of the case, the condition of the child and of his parents, if any, the residence and trade of the proposed master and other points; and subsequently, if the child is less than 14 years of age, a medical certificate of fitness is obtained.

The person to whom a child is bound must be a 'housekeeper or assessed to the poor-rate in his own name'—not a journeyman or 'person not carrying on trade or business on his own account,' a person under 21 years of age, or a married woman. The place of business at which the apprentice has to live and work must not be more than 30 miles from the place where the child is residing at the time of apprenticeship. If the apprentice is above the age of 16, and not by reason of deformity, or other such cause, unfit for work, no premium is given except clothing. In other cases the premium is given part in money, part in clothing; and the former is payable, one moiety at the binding, the remainder after the first year of apprenticeship. The term of apprenticeship is not more than eight years. The consent of the person to be bound apprentice, if not more than 14 years of age, has to be obtained, and if he be not more than 16 years of age, the consent of the parent or guardian is, with some exceptions, required. The apprenticeship is by indenture.

The master has to teach the trade or business agreed upon, and has to provide proper food, lodging and clothing, and in case of sickness or accident, 'adequate medical or surgical assistance'; he must arrange for suitable religious instruction being given, according to the creed of the apprentice; after 17, the apprentice may be paid such wages as the Guardians may stipulate. If the terms of the indenture are transgressed by the master, or he becomes bankrupt, the indenture is cancelled.

Apprenticeship to sea service by the Guardians. (6) Apprenticeship to sea service.—The Guardians may apprentice boys by indenture to masters and owners of ships.[1] The indenture must be attested by two justices, who shall ascertain that the boy has consented, that he is sufficiently healthy, strong, and that he is bound to a proper person.

Guardians may also pay the expenses of boys who, or whose parents, are in receipt of Poor Law relief, in going to the nearest port to be examined, and they may pay for their outfit.[2] There are a large number of training and coastguard ships at which boys are sent by the Guardians for entry in H.M. naval service.

Supervision of apprentices and servants placed out by the Guardians. The Guardians are bound to keep a register of those under the age of 16 whom they have placed as apprentices or in service, and to cause them while under that age and in the same service to be

[1] Merchant Shipping Act, August 10, 1854 (17 & 18 Vict., c. 104), s. 141, etc.
[2] 39 & 40 Vict., c. 61, s. 28.

visited twice a year by a relieving officer, who reports to the Guardians on their food and treatment.[1]

Furthermore, the Guardians, or the managers of a district school, may employ a visitor to report upon the condition, treatment, and conduct of any child under the age of 16 who has gone into service from the workhouse or the school.[2]

The conditions required in cases in which apprenticeship fees are paid from charitable funds are similar to those required in the cases dealt with by Boards of Guardians. The almoner will probably have little difficulty in securing skilled advice so far as it may be necessary, and suitable forms, such, for instance, as those used by the East London Apprenticing Fund.

Apprenticeship by charitable persons.

Since 1879 the Guardians have, with the consent of the Local Government Board, been empowered to subscribe towards any association or society for aiding girls and boys in service, or towards any other asylum or institution which appears to the Guardians to be calculated to render useful aid in the administration of the relief of the poor.[3]

As regards servants placed out by the Guardians, the Metropolitan Association for Befriending Young Servants, Buckingham Street, Strand, W.C., is of the greatest use. The Local Government Board in their Annual Report[4] for 1887–8, state that 'a considerable proportion of the girls who go from the Poor Law Schools of the Metropolis into domestic service are placed by the Guardians under the supervision of the Metropolitan Association for Befriending Young Servants.' In the report of the Association for the year 1891 the number of girls supervised by the Association during the year was 3,392, and of these 2,504 were from the District and Separate Poor Law Schools of the Metropolis. Of the 3,392 girls referred to, 1,743 were classed as 'good,' 680 as 'fair,' 243 as 'unsatisfactory,' and 35 as 'bad.' As regards the remainder, 5 are dead, 53 were unfit for service, 86 refused to be visited, 131 were lost sight of or not traced; 38 have emigrated or married, 131 are with their relatives, 186 are in training homes, and 77 are not as yet reported on.

The M.A.B.Y.S.

The almoner is strongly recommended, in dealing with the many cases in which assistance can be given by way of training for service or obtaining a place for an elder daughter, to co-operate with such societies as the M.A.B.Y.S.

For assisting children, then, as these six sections indicate, the Guardians have almost unlimited powers.

Before considering the part which charity should take in dealing with the cases of widows, we may refer to the liabilities of

[1] 14 & 15 Vict., c. 11, ss. 3, 4, and 5. [2] 39 & 40 Vict., c. 61, s. 33.
[3] 42 & 43 Vict., c. 54, s. 10 (*see* p. cvi.).
[4] Seventeenth Annual Report, p. lii. 1887–8.

masters, and the supervision which the Guardians exercise over servants and apprentices. The survey of the powers in this department will then be complete.

XXXVI.—Protection of Infants and Young People: Liability of Masters.

Liabilities of masters and servants.

Besides the provision made for the supervision and care of apprentices or servants placed out by the Guardians, there are some general provisions, greatly strengthened by recent legislation, for the prevention and punishment of neglect in the cases of infants, children, and young persons. The almoner will very likely come across some such cases.

Any person legally liable as master or mistress to provide necessary food, clothing, lodging, to an apprentice or servant who shall wilfully and without lawful excuse refuse or neglect to do so, or shall unlawfully and maliciously do or cause to be done any bodily harm so that the life of such apprentice or servant shall be endangered, or the health of such apprentice or servant shall have been or shall be likely to be permanently endangered, is liable, on conviction, to three years' penal servitude, or imprisonment for any term not exceeding two years, with or without hard labour.[1]

If complaint be made to two justices of any such neglect as this, or of any bodily injury inflicted on any person under 16, the circumstances of which amount to a felony, or the attempt to commit a felony, they may require the Guardians to prosecute; and the Guardians will 'pay the costs reasonably and properly incurred by them out of the common fund of the Union.'[2]

Further, a master who, being legally liable to provide for his apprentice necessary food, clothing, medical aid, or lodging, wilfully and without lawful excuse refuses or neglects to provide the same, whereby the health of the apprentice is or is likely to be seriously or permanently injured, is liable, on conviction, to a penalty of not exceeding £20, or imprisonment for a term not exceeding six months, with or without hard labour.[3]

The prevention of 'baby farming.'

There is another legal provision worthy of note in this connection. No person may retain or receive for hire or reward more than one infant, and in case of twins more than two infants, under the age of one year, for the purpose of nursing or maintaining them apart from their parents for a longer period than 24 hours, except in a registered house.[4]

The Act does not extend to relations or guardians, nor to public institutions, etc. The local authority (in London the County Council) are empowered, after careful inquiry as to fitness,

---

[1] 21 & 25 Vict., c. 100, s. 26.   [2] 24 & 25 Vict., c. 100, s. 73.

[3] 38 & 39 Vict., c. 86, ss. 6 & 10.   [4] 35 & 36 Vict., c. 38.

to register houses and persons for the above purpose (registration gratis—renewable annually), and from time to time to make bye-laws for fixing the number of infants which may be received into each such house. It has been the practice in London to make a special bye-law upon each individual application. Offenders are liable to six months' imprisonment with hard labour, or a fine of £5.

When, on the trial of any offence under the Criminal Law Amendment Act 1885, it is proved to the satisfaction of the Court *Girls under 16.* that the seduction or prostitution of any girl under the age of 16 has been caused, encouraged, or favoured by her father, mother, guardian, master, or mistress, the Court may divest such person of all authority over her, and appoint a guardian for her until she is 21, and appoint, if necessary, a new guardian from time to time.[1]

But during the last session of Parliament (1894) has been passed the most stringent Act for the punishment for ill-treatment and neglect of children, a consolidation of Acts adopted in 1889 and 1894.[2] The following are the first seven sections:

'Cruelty to Children.

'1.—(1) If any person over the age of sixteen years who has the custody, *Punishment for cruelty to children.* charge, or care of any child under the age of sixteen years, wilfully assaults, ill-treats, neglects, abandons, or exposes such child, or causes or procures such child to be assaulted, ill-treated, neglected, abandoned, or exposed in a manner likely to cause such child unnecessary suffering, or injury to its health (including injury to or loss of sight, or hearing, or limb, or organ of the body, and any mental derangement), that person shall be guilty of a misdemeanor; and

'(a) on conviction on indictment, shall be liable, at the discretion of the court, to a fine not exceeding one hundred pounds, or alternatively, or in default of payment of such fine, or in addition thereto, to imprisonment, with or without hard labour, for any term not exceeding two years ; and

'(b) on summary conviction shall be liable, at the discretion of the court, to a fine not exceeding twenty-five pounds, or alternatively, or in default of payment of such fine, or in addition thereto, to imprisonment, with or without hard labour, for any term not exceeding six months.

'(2) A person may be convicted of an offence under this section either on indictment or by a court of summary jurisdiction notwithstanding the death of the child in respect of whom the offence is committed.

'(3) If it is proved that a person indicted under this section was interested in any sum of money accruable or payable in the event of the death of the child, and had knowledge that such sum of money was accruing or becoming payable, the court, in its discretion, may

'(a) increase the amount of the fine under this section so that the fine does not exceed two hundred pounds ; or

'(b) in lieu of awarding any other penalty under this section, sentence the person indicted to penal servitude for any term not exceeding five years.

'(4) A person shall be deemed to be interested in a sum of money under this section if he has any share in or any benefit from the payment of that money, though he is not a person to whom it is legally payable.

'(5) An offence under this section is in this Act referred to as an offence of cruelty.

---

[1] 48 & 49 Vict., c. 69, s. 12.
[2] Prevention of Cruelty to Children Act 1894 (57 & 58 Vict., c. 51).

' *Restrictions on Employment of Children.*[1]

Restrictions on employment of children.

' 2. If any person—

(*a*) causes or procures any child, being a boy under the age of fourteen years, or being a girl under the age of sixteen years, or, having the custody, charge, or care of any such child, allows that child, to be in any street, premises, or place for the purpose of begging or receiving alms, or of inducing the giving of alms, whether under the pretence of singing, playing, performing, offering anything for sale, or otherwise ; or

' (*b*) causes or procures any child, being a boy under the age of fourteen years, or being a girl under the age of sixteen years, or, having the custody, charge, or care of any such child, allows that child, to be in any street, or in any premises licensed for the sale of any intoxicating liquor, other than premises licensed according to law for public entertainments, for the purpose of singing, playing, or performing for profit, or offering anything for sale, between 9 P.M. and 6 A.M.; or

' (*c*) causes or procures any child under the age of eleven years, or, having the custody, charge, or care of any such child, allows that child, to be at any time in any street, or in any premises licensed for the sale of any intoxicating liquor, or in premises licensed according to law for public entertainments, or in any circus or other place of public amusement to which the public are admitted by payment, for the purpose of singing, playing, or performing for profit, or offering anything for sale ; or

' (*d*) causes or procures any child under the age of sixteen years, or, having the custody, charge, or care of any such child, allows that child, to be in any place for the purpose of being trained as an acrobat, contortionist, or circus performer, or of being trained for any exhibition or performance which in its nature is dangerous,[2]

that person shall, on summary conviction, be liable, at the discretion of the court, to a fine not exceeding twenty-five pounds, or alternatively, or in default of payment of such fine, or in addition thereto, to imprisonment, with or without hard labour, for any term not exceeding three months.

' Provided that—

' (i.) This section shall not apply in the case of any occasional sale or entertainment the net proceeds of which are wholly applied for the benefit of any school or to any charitable object, if such sale or entertainment is held elsewhere than in premises which are licensed for the sale of any intoxicating liquor but not licensed according to law for public entertainments, or if, in the case of a sale or entertainment held in any such premises as aforesaid, a special exemption from the provisions of this section has been granted in writing under the hands of two justices of the peace ; and

' (ii.) Any local authority may, if they think it necessary or desirable so to do, from time to time by byelaw extend or restrict the hours mentioned in paragraph (*b*) of this section, either on every day or on any specified day or days of the week, and either as to the whole of their district or as to any specified area therein ; and

' (iii.) Paragraphs (*c*) and (*d*) of this section shall not apply in any case in respect of which a licence granted under this Act is in force, so far as that licence extends ; and

' (iv.) Paragraph (*d*) of this section shall not apply in the case of a person who is the parent or legal guardian of a child, and himself trains the child.

Licences for employment of children.

' 3.—(1) A petty sessional court, or in Scotland the School Board, may, notwithstanding anything in this Act, grant a licence for such time and during such hours of the day, and subject to such restrictions and conditions as the court or board think fit, for any child exceeding seven years of age,—

' (*a*) to take part in any entertainment or series of entertainments to take place in premises licensed according to law for public entertainments, or in any circus or other place of public amusement as aforesaid ; or

' (*b*) to be trained as aforesaid ; or for both purposes ;

---

[1] *Cf.* Vagrancy Act, p. lxvi.
[2] *Cf.* Limitations on the employment of children, p. cxiii.

if satisfied of the fitness of the child for the purpose, and if it is shown to their satisfaction that proper provision has been made to secure the health and kind treatment of the children taking part in the entertainment or series of entertainments or being trained as aforesaid, and the court or board may, upon sufficient cause, vary, add to, or rescind any such licence.

'Any such licence shall be sufficient protection to all persons acting under or in accordance with the same.

'(2) A Secretary of State may assign to any inspector appointed under section sixty-seven of the Factory and Workshop Act 1878, specially and in addition to any other usual duties, the duty of seeing whether the restrictions and conditions of any licence under this section are duly complied with, and any such inspector shall have the same power to enter, inspect, and examine any place of public entertainment at which the employment of a child is for the time being licensed under this section as an inspector has to enter, inspect, and examine a factory or workshop under section sixty-eight of the same Act. **41 & 42 Vict., c. 16.**

'(3) Where any person applies for a licence under this section he shall, at least seven days before making the application, give notice thereof to the chief officer of police for the district in which the licence is to take effect, and that officer may appear or instruct some person to appear before the authority hearing the application, and show cause why the licence should not be granted, and the authority to whom the application is made shall not grant the same unless they are satisfied that notice has been properly so given.

'(4) Where a licence is granted under this section to any person, that person shall, not less than ten days after the granting of the licence, cause a copy thereof to be sent to the inspector of factories and workshops acting for the district in which the licence is to take effect, and if he fails to cause such copy to be sent, shall be liable on summary conviction to a fine not exceeding five pounds.

'(5) Nothing in this or in the last preceding section shall affect the provisions of the Elementary Education Act 1876, or the Education (Scotland) Act 1878. **39 & 40 Vict., c. 79; 41 & 42 Vict., c. 78.**

'*Arrest of Offender and Provision for Safety of Children.*'

'4.—(1) Any constable may take into custody, without warrant, any person— **Power to take offenders into custody.**

'(*a*) who within view of such constable commits an offence under this Act, or any of the offences mentioned in the Schedule to this Act, where the name and residence of such person are unknown to such constable, and cannot be ascertained by such constable ; or

'(*b*) who has committed, or who he has reason to believe has committed, any offence of cruelty within the meaning of this Act, or any of the offences mentioned in the Schedule to this Act, if he has reasonable ground for believing that such person will abscond, or if the name and address of such person are unknown to and cannot be ascertained by the constable.

'(2) Where a constable arrests any person without warrant in pursuance of this section, the inspector or constable in charge of the station to which such person is conveyed shall, unless in his belief the release of such person on bail would tend to defeat the ends of justice, or to cause injury or danger to the child against whom the offence is alleged to have been committed, release the person arrested on his entering into such a recognisance, with or without sureties, as may in his judgment be required to secure the attendance of such person upon the hearing of the charge.

'It will be noted that the procedure of the Act, sections 4, 5, and 6, is extended to other Acts and even further. The Schedule here referred to is as follows : –

'Any offence under sections 27 [regarding the abandonment or exposure of children under the age of 2, so as to endanger life or injure health permanently], 55 [regarding abduction], or 56 [regarding child stealing] of the Offences against the Person Act 1861, and any offence against any child under the age of 16 years under sections 43 [respecting aggravated assaults] and 52 [indecent assaults] of that Act (24 & 25 Vict., c. 100).

'Any offence under the Children's Dangerous Performances Act 1879' (42 & 43 Vict., c. 34), and lastly,

'Any other offence involving bodily injury to a child under the age of 16 years.' With regard to these Acts, *see* also p. lix.

Detention of child in place of safety.

' 5.—(1) A constable may take to a place of safety any child in respect of whom an offence under paragraph (a) of section two of this Act has been committed, or in respect of whom an offence of cruelty within the meaning of this Act, or any of the offences mentioned in the Schedule to this Act, has been, or there is reason to believe has been, committed.

' (2) A child so taken to a place of safety, and also any child under the age of sixteen years who seeks refuge in a place of safety, may there be detained until it can be brought before a court of summary jurisdiction, and that court may make such order as is mentioned in the next following sub-section, or may cause the child to be dealt with as circumstances may admit and require until the charge made against any person in respect of any offence as aforesaid with regard to the child has been determined, by the committal for trial, or conviction, or discharge of such person.

' (3) Where it appears to a court of summary jurisdiction or any justice that an offence of cruelty within the meaning of this Act, or any of the offences mentioned in the Schedule to this Act, has been committed in the case of any child that is brought before such court or justice, and that the health or safety of the child will be endangered unless an order is made under this sub-section, the court or justice may, without prejudice to any other power under this Act, make such order as circumstances require for the care and detention of the child until a reasonable time has elapsed for a charge to be made against some person for having committed the offence, and, if a charge is made against any person within that time, until the charge has been determined by the committal for trial or conviction or discharge of that person, and any such order may be carried out notwithstanding that any person claims the custody of the child.

'(4) Boards of guardians, and, in Scotland, parochial boards, shall provide for the reception of children brought to a workhouse in pursuance of this Act, and where the place of safety to which a constable takes a child is a workhouse the master shall receive the child into the workhouse if there is suitable accommodation therein for the same, and shall detain the child until the case is determined, and any expenses incurred in respect of the child shall be deemed to be expenses incurred in the relief of the poor.

Disposal of child by order of court.

' 6.—(1) Where a person having the custody, charge, or care of a child under the age of sixteen years has been—

' (a) convicted of committing in respect of such child an offence of cruelty within the meaning of this Act, or any of the offences mentioned in the Schedule to this Act ; or

' (b) committed for trial for any such offence ; or

' (c) bound over to keep the peace towards such child,

by any court, that court either at the time when the person is so convicted, committed for trial, or bound over, and without requiring any new proceedings to be instituted for the purpose, or at any other time, and also any petty sessional court before which any person may bring the case, if satisfied on inquiry that it is expedient so to deal with the child, order that the child be taken out of the custody of the person so convicted, committed for trial, or bound over, and be committed to the custody of a relation of the child, or some other fit person named by the court (such relation or other person being willing to undertake such custody), until it attains the age of sixteen years, or for any shorter period, and may of its own motion or on the application of any person from time to time by order renew, vary, and revoke any such order ; but no order shall be made under this section unless a parent of the child has been convicted of or committed for trial for the offence, or is under committal for trial, for having been or has been proved to have been party or privy to the offence, or has been bound over to keep the peace towards such child.

' (2) Every order under this section shall be in writing, and any such order may be made by the court in the absence of the child ; and the consent of any person to undertake the custody of a child in pursuance of any such order shall be proved in such manner as the court may think sufficient to bind him

' (3) Where an order is made under this section in respect of a person who has been committed for trial, then if that person is acquitted of the charge, or if the charge is dismissed for want of prosecution, the order shall forthwith be void except with regard to anything that may have been lawfully done under it.

'(4) A Secretary of State in England, and in Scotland the Secretary for Scotland, and in Ireland the Lord Lieutenant of Ireland, may at any time in his discretion discharge a child from the custody of any person to whose custody it is committed in pursuance of this section, either absolutely or on such conditions as such Secretary of State, Secretary, or Lord Lieutenant approves, and may, if he thinks fit, make rules in relation to children so committed to the custody of any person, and to the duties of such persons with respect to such children.

'(5) A Secretary of State, in any case where it appears to him to be for the benefit of a child who has been committed to the custody of any person in pursuance of this section, may empower such person to procure the emigration of the child, but, except with such authority, no person to whose custody a child is so committed shall procure its emigration.

'7.—(1) Any person to whose custody a child is committed under this Act shall, whilst the order is in force, have the like control over the child as if he were its parent, and shall be responsible for its maintenance, and the child shall continue in the custody of such person, notwithstanding that it is claimed by its parent.

Maintenance of child when committed to custody of any person under order of court.

'(2) Any court having power so to commit a child shall have power to make the like orders on the parent of the child to contribute to its maintenance during such period as aforesaid as if the child were detained under the Industrial Schools Acts, but the limit on the amount of the weekly sum which the parent of a child may be required, under this section, to contribute to its maintenance shall be one pound a week instead of the limit fixed by the Industrial Schools Acts.

'(3) Any such order may be made on the complaint or application of the person to whose custody the child is for the time being committed, and either at the time when the order for the child's committal to custody is made, or subsequently, and the sums contributed by the parent shall be paid to such person as the court may name, and be applied for the maintenance of the child.

'(4) If a person fails to pay any sum payable by him in pursuance of any such order, he may be dealt with in like manner as if the sum were due from him in pursuance of an order under the Bastardy Law Amendment Act 1872, or in Scotland were a sum decerned for aliment, or in Ireland were a sum ordered to be paid by him under the Summary Jurisdiction (Ireland) Acts.

35 & 36 Vict., c. 65.

'(5) Where an order under this Act to commit a child to the custody of some relation or other person is made in respect of a person who has been committed for trial for an offence, the court shall not have power to order the parent of the child to contribute to its maintenance prior to the trial of that person.'

Three definitions in the Act may be quoted :—

(1) 'Street' includes 'any highway or other public place, whether a thoroughfare or not.'

(2) 'The provisions of the Act relating to the parent of a child shall apply to the step-parent of the child, and to any person cohabiting with the parent of the child, and the expression "parent," when used in relation to a child, includes guardian and any person who is by law liable to maintain the child.'

(3) ' Any person who is the parent of a child shall be presumed to have the custody of the child ; and any person to whose charge a child is committed by its parent shall be presumed to have charge of the child ; and

'Any other person having actual possession or control of a child shall be presumed to have the care of the child.'[1]

The Guardians may pay and charge to the union funds ' the reasonable costs and expenses of any proceedings which they have directed to be taken under this Act in regard to the assault,

[1] Sec. 23.

ill-treatment, neglect, abandonment, or exposure of any child.'[1] 'The Act shall apply in the case of a parent who, being without means to maintain a child, fails to provide for its maintenance under the Acts relating to the relief of the poor, in like manner as if the parent had otherwise neglected the child.'[2] Therefore want of means is no excuse for neglect, since to relieve the destitute the Poor Law was established.

Children are also protected in another way. By the Children's Dangerous Performances Act 1879, above referred to—

'Any person who shall cause any child under the age of fourteen years to take part in any public exhibition or performance whereby, in the opinion of a court of summary jurisdiction, the life or limbs of such child shall be endangered, and the parent or guardian, or any person having the custody, of such child, who shall aid or abet the same, shall severally be guilty of an offence against this Act, and shall on summary conviction be liable for each offence to a penalty not exceeding ten pounds.'[3]

If an accident causing actual bodily harm occurs under these circumstances the employer is liable to be indicted as having committed an assault, and compensation not exceeding twenty pounds may be awarded on conviction.

Both the Metropolitan and the City police, it may be mentioned, have been instructed in all cases which come to their knowledge, in which children are treated with cruelty, either by their parents or others, whether witnessed by or reported to the police, to notify the particulars at once to the London Society for the Prevention of Cruelty to Children, and the police are to afford every information and assistance in their power. Also when children are apprehended under the Vagrant Act the Society is to be at once informed of the arrest, and on application its officer will be permitted to bail the child, to take charge of it, and to produce it at the police court at the hearing of the case.[4]

XXXVII.—Assistance of Widows and Children.

The part to be taken by Poor Law and Charity in assisting widows.

The legal provisions mentioned in Section XXXI. and the following sections show that the cases of persons left destitute at widowhood may fairly be left to the Guardians. Improvidence must carry its own penalty with it, and, if the Poor Law schools do their part in depauperising the children, little can be said against the conditions of assistance, which are comparatively lenient. The Guardians in some Unions relieve widows with out-relief sometimes at a low and apparently insufficient rate, and sometimes at the high scale of 9s. a week. In other Unions the widow is assisted either in the house, or by the admission to a Poor Law school of so many of her children as she may be unable to support.[5] Whatever practice is adopted, it is

---

[1] Sec. 20.   [2] Sec. 23 (2).   [3] 42 & 43 Vict., c. 34 (1879).
[4] Police Order, Metropolitan Police, March 25, 1889.
[5] With regard to non-resident relief to widows, *see* pp. xxxiii. & xxxv.

unwise for charity to supplement Poor Law relief. Generally its effect is to withdraw from charity, and to waste, a large sum of money which, well applied, would be of great use in cases in which charity should rightly undertake the whole responsibility. Clergy and almoners often say they have so many cases to deal with that they cannot do much for any, and that they have no money to spare for cases requiring a few pounds. They often relieve Poor Law cases, and distribute their money so that the participators in it may be numerous. They thus injure many by insufficient casual aid and may really assist none. Such charity is but ' saving the rates '—it is so much added to the loaves and shillings which the Guardians might equally well have paid. It degrades charity to the level of Poor Law relief, and assimilates it to it. As a general rule, therefore, the practice should be avoided. The cases of widows in which the Guardians take some of the children into the schools, are exceptions. Sometimes the widow may be able to get her own living with help which the Guardians (see p. xxxv.) cannot legally give. By intervention in such an instance charity may do a lasting service, especially if some provident plan can be arranged for the applicant's old age.

Widows with young families may be roughly divided into two broad classes:—(1) Where the mother is weak in mind or body, and consequently will always need help in some form until the children can earn money. This class may fairly be left to the Poor Law, in the absence of any special claim arising out of the husband's merits. (2) Where the mother is a person of energy and resource, whom temporary help will enable to support the family. Such a case should be assisted by charity. Special consideration should be given to the antecedents of the husband, though the character of these antecedents should not be taken as a final test. Then every direct and indirect mode of assisting has to be resorted to, such as is indicated in the case quoted on p. xcv., and in the following :—

This case had been previously known to the Committee, and had been assisted by it between two and three years before. When it was referred as a School Board case, the family consisted of a widow with nine children, the three eldest of whom were daughters in service, but not earning enough to assist their mother much. One girl of 14 was in an orphanage. The mother and her five remaining children, aged 16, 12½, 10, 5, and 3, were all living in one small room, almost entirely dependent on the earnings of the one aged 16, a boy who gained 9s. a week. The ill-health of the mother prevented her going out to work. Nearly everything the family possessed was pawned ; but, though their distress was very great, they had never applied for parish relief. The Committee placed the girl aged 12½ in a Training Home for Young Servants, from whence, when she is 13, she will be put into a situation. The girl of 10 they tried to place in a school, but her health not being sufficiently good to pass the medical examination required she was sent to a sea-side Convalescent Home for three months, as a lengthened stay at the sea-side was said to be the only thing to prevent her becoming a permanent invalid. The child of five was enabled to attend school. Sufficient things were redeemed from pawn to restore the family to comparative comfort, and some needlework obtained for the mother, who was thus enabled to add a few shillings to the weekly income.

Typical case of charitable relief to a widow.

'Mrs. L. came to us in the spring of last year, whose husband had died six months before. She had seven children to bring up, two of them twin babies, born after her husband's death. The problem was, how could she be helped? Fortunately, her relations had come forward and helped her over her confinement, and one of them had adopted a boy age three, but they could do no more. The first thing that we did was to place three of the little boys in good schools; two of them were admitted to the Shaftesbury Homes, and are now doing well at Bisley, and the third is boarded-out in a cottage home at Harrow, through the Waifs and Strays Society. Emma, the eldest girl, age 14, began to learn artificial flower making, and is now earning a few shillings weekly; it is such a comfort to her mother to have her at home that we did not urge domestic service in this case, as we usually do for girls at her age. Then we had to think of work for the mother, which on account of her babies must be home work. She thought if she could have a wringing machine she could take in washing, so with the help of the Widow's Friend Society we obtained this, and she is now working up a connection, but, seeing that her twins require a good deal of her attention, we have obtained from friends interested in her two shillings a week to help towards her rent, until she is able to go alone. A lady visits her regularly in a friendly way, and tells us that her home is always clean and tidy, and her children well cared for. In the summer, finding Mrs. L. and her babies ailing, we sent them to the seaside for a few weeks, and altogether we have spent over £10 on this family. Has it not been well spent in keeping a respectable woman off the parish, and giving her and her children a chance of becoming independent?'

Out-relief, Poor Law assistance, and education.

When the parent of a child between 5 and 14 years of age, or the child, receives relief out of the workhouse, by way of weekly and other continuing allowance,[1] it is a condition of relief that, subject to reasonable excuses,[2] the child should attend school, if the child has not reached the third standard (1876), or is not entitled to take full time employment, or is required by the bye-laws of the School Board to attend school.[3] The Guardians in such cases are not precluded from allowing additional relief to the parent in consequence of the reduction of the parent's income by loss of the child's earnings. They may also pay for clothing for the child's attendance at school.[4] See also below (Section XXXIX.) as to the School Board.

XXXVIII.—SUBSCRIPTIONS TO INSTITUTIONS BY 'GUARDIANS.

The question is frequently asked whether the Guardians can pay subscriptions towards institutions of which they make use, and if so, to what institutions; and it is worth while to quote the sections of the Acts on the subject as they stand, though they include several classes of cases besides those already referred to.

'By 14 & 15 Vict., c. 105, s. 4, the Guardians of any union or parish may, with the consent of the Poor Law Board, pay out of the common fund of such union, or, in the case of a parish, out of the funds in hand of such Guardians, any sum of money as an annual subscription towards the support and maintenance of any

[1] 39 & 40 Vict., c. 79, s. 40 (1876).
[2] For what are reasonable excuses, see 'Summary of Law,' &c., published by the London School Board, p. cviii.
[3] Bye-laws cannot be made with regard to children above the age of 13, therefore this last proviso will only apply to children under the age of 13.
[4] See on the whole question, 'The Elementary Education Acts,' 1870 to 1880, by Hugh Owen. Knight & Co., 1881. See especially pp. 290 and 319.

public hospital or infirmary for the reception of the sick, diseased, disabled, or wounded persons, or persons suffering from any permanent or natural infirmity.

'The provisions of 14 & 15 Vict., c. 105, s. 4, shall extend to authorise the Guardians, with such consent as is therein mentioned, to subscribe towards any asylum or institution for blind persons, or deaf and dumb persons, or for persons suffering from any permanent or natural infirmity, or towards any association or society for aiding such persons, or for providing nurses, or for aiding girls or boys in service, or towards any other asylum or institution which appears to the Guardians, with such consent as aforesaid, to be calculated to render useful aid in the administration of the relief of the poor.[1]

'Provided always, that nothing herein contained shall authorise any subscription to any asylum or institution unless the Local Government Board be satisfied that the paupers under the Guardians have or could have assistance therein in case of necessity.'[2]

XXXIX.—The School Board and the Education of Children.

The School Board (Victoria Embankment) consists of 50 members, elected triennially in numbers varying from four to seven from the eleven electoral divisions of the City, Chelsea, Finsbury, Greenwich, Hackney, East and West Lambeth, Marylebone, Southwark, Tower Hamlets, Westminster. The local work is entrusted to Divisional and Sub-divisional Committees, under whom serve paid superintendents of visitors. Education is free[3] in the schools of the London School Board.

The Education Act of 1876 declares that—'It shall be the duty of the parent of every child (between the ages of 5 and 14) to cause such child to receive efficient elementary instruction in reading, General responsibilities of parents in regard to the education of their children.

[1] 42 & 43 Vict., c. 54, s. 10. Glen's Archbold, p. 82.
[2] It is convenient to refer here to the power of Boards of Guardians, to contract with the proprietors of certain establishments, to send paupers to them. By 12 Vict., c. 13, ss. 1 and 2, the Local Government Board are required from time to time, as they shall see occasion, to 'issue rules, orders, and regulations for the management and government of any house or establishment wherein any poor person shall be lodged, boarded, or maintained, for hire or remuneration, under any contract or agreement entered into by the proprietor, manager, or superintendent, or on his beha'f, with any guardians . . . in like manner and to the same extent as they are empowered to do in the case of any workhouse belonging to any union or parish.' But this does not apply to lunatic asylums or 'to any hospital, infirmary, school, or other institution supported by public subscriptions, and maintained for purposes of charity only.' The Board can also regulate the contracts made with such proprietors and inspect their establishments. The Board have issued an order containing, in accordance with the above Act, 'regulations for seaside infirmaries for scrofulous cases'; and contracts have been entered into with two establishments at Margate, and one at Rottingdean. (Cf. Glen, Poor Law Statutes, p. 904, and Orders, p. 267.) The order is addressed to, amongst others, the 'several Unions and separate Parishes of the Metropolis.'
[3] Elementary Education Act 1891, 54 & 55 Vict., c. 56.

writing, and arithmetic.' To ensure the fulfilment of this duty, there are safeguards against the child being employed, unless sufficiently instructed, *i.e.* unless he has passed a certain 'standard,' and there are penalties against the parent if the child does not go to school.[1] The following is taken from a paper published by the London School Board. It puts the requirements of the Board very clearly, and as the compulsory education of the children is a domestic question, sometimes a domestic difficulty, in the households of the poor, and is frequently put forward as a grievance or a claim for help, the almoner should know what the requirements are.

' District of the School Board for London.

' *Elementary Education Acts of* 1870, 1873, 1876, 1880, 1891, & 1893.

' I.—Summary of the Law relating to the Attendance at School of Children between 5 and 14 years of age, and to the Employment of such Children.

'*A. As to children between 5 and 13.*

' A child between 5 and 13 years of age must attend a certified efficient school during the whole time for which such school is open.

' Exceptions : —

' (i.) A child between 11 and 13 years of age is not required to attend school for more than five attendances in each week, if such child shall be shown to the satisfaction of the School Board to be beneficially and necessarily employed, and shall have received a certificate from one of Her Majesty's Inspectors that it has passed the *Fourth* Standard.

' (ii.) A child between 11 and 13 years of age is not required to attend school at all, if such child shall have received a certificate from one of Her Majesty's Inspectors that it has passed the *Sixth* Standard.

' The following are reasonable excuses for the non-attendance of a child at school:—

' (*a*) That the child is under efficient instruction in some other manner.

' (*b*) That the child is prevented from attending school by sickness or any unavoidable cause.

' (*c*) That there is no public elementary school open which the child can attend within two miles.

' The parent, or guardian, of any child who ought to attend but

---

[1] ' " Parent " includes guardian and everyone who is liable to maintain or has the custody of any child.'

does not attend school, is liable upon conviction to a penalty not exceeding, with the costs, five shillings for each offence.

'Moreover, the employer[1] of any child who ought to attend but does not attend school, is liable to a penalty not exceeding forty shillings for each offence.

'*B. As to children between 13 and 14.*

' No person, parent or other, may take into his employment any child between 13 and 14 years of age unless such child (*a*) shall have obtained a certificate that he has passed the *Fourth* Standard, *or* (*b*) shall have made 250 attendances in not more than two schools during each year for five preceding years, whether consecutive or not, *or* (*c*) shall be attending school in accordance with the provisions of the Factory Acts.

'The employer of a child between 13 and 14 years of age, who has not satisfied one of these two conditions, is liable to a penalty not exceeding forty shillings: and if such child is habitually absent from school, the parent is liable to successive penalties of five shillings each.'

The second part of the summary from which we quote deals with the payment of fees, and the third with the attendance of blind or deaf children. These points are set forth more conveniently for our purpose in the 'Byelaws,' etc., of the Board, which explain the Board's procedure in this matter.

II.—The Payment of Fees.

With regard to the payment of fees the law stands thus, as set forth in the 'Byelaws, Arrangements, and Code of Instructions' of the School Board for London (March 15, 1894) :—

' A parent may be summoned to a "Notice B" meeting in consequence of the non-attendance of his child at school, and, if attending, or proposing to attend, a non-Board school where fees are charged, may plead as a reason his inability to pay the fees.'

Payment of School fees by Guardians of the Poor.

'(1) *Cases of parents who are non-paupers.*

'A parent (not being a pauper) of any child [between the ages of 5 and 14, or in the case of a deaf child between the ages of 5 and 16, or in the case of a blind child between the ages of 7 and 16] "who is unable by reason of poverty to pay the ordinary fee for such child at a public elementary school, or any part of such fee, may apply to the Guardians having jurisdiction in the parish in which he resides ; and it shall be the duty of such Guardians, if satisfied of such inability, to pay the said fee. not exceeding threepence per week, or such part thereof as he is, in the opinion of the Guardians, so unable to pay." [Elementary Education Act 1876, Section 10.]

'In the above cases the parents should be informed that application for the payment of the fees must be made to the Guardians of the Poor, and the cases should be reported to the Correspondent of the non-Board School which may

---

[1] ' Employer' includes 'a parent who employs his child by way of trade or for the purposes of gain.'

have been selected. A list of the children should also be forwarded by the Divisional Superintendent to the Clerk of the Guardians on Form No. 32.

'(2) *Cases of parents who are out-door paupers.*

' " Where relief out of the workhouse is given by the Guardians or their order, by way of weekly or other weekly continuing allowance," to the parent of any child between the ages of 5 and 13, or in the case of a deaf child between the ages of 5 and 16, or in the case of a blind child between the ages of 7 and 16, the Guardians are bound to make it " a condition for the continuance of such relief that elementary education in reading, writing, and arithmetic shall be provided for such child, and the Guardians shall give such further relief (if any) as may be necessary for the purpose." [Elementary Education Act 1876, Section 40, and Elementary Education Act 1880, Section 5.]

' The parents in all such cases should therefore be referred to the Guardians ; and the Divisional Superintendent must further report such cases to the Correspondent of the non-Board School which may have been selected.

' If, however, the Divisional Superintendent has reason to believe that " further relief " is not given for the payment of the fees, he is to represent the facts to the Guardians, and, in the event of the Guardians refusing to make provision for the payment of the fees, to report the matter to the School Accommodation and Attendance Committee.

' Special attention is to be given to the attendance of the children whose fees are being paid in non-Board Schools by the Guardians of the Poor.

' NOTE.—With reference to the payment of fees by Guardians of the Poor under Sections 10 and 40 of the Act of 1876, the Local Government Board, in a circular dated September 17, 1891, relating to the Free Education Act, state as follows :—

' " The provisions of the Act are chiefly of interest to the Guardians in so far as they may affect the payment by them of school fees. With regard to this, the Board direct me to point out that the Act does not repeal either Section 10 of the Elementary Education Act 1876, as to the payment of the school fees of children of parents who are not paupers, or Section 40 of the same Act, relating to relief for the payment of the school fees of pauper children in certain cases where outdoor relief is given. The payment of school fees under Section 10, or the granting of further relief under Section 40, to enable school fees not exceeding 3d. a week to be paid, must not be made or granted on condition of the child attending any public elementary school other than such as may be selected by the parent, nor refused because the child attends, or does not attend, any particular public elementary school. Although, therefore, where a child attends a free school, or is not required to pay a fee at any fee-charging school which he attends, the duty of the Guardians under these sections will cease with respect to him, their duty will remain the same as before the passing of the new Act with respect to any child who can only attend the school on payment of a fee." '

The addresses of the School Board Offices in each division are entered in the local lists.

School Management Committees. ' The School Board may, if it think fit, from time to time delegate any of their powers under this Act (the Education Act of 1870), except the power of raising money ; and, in particular, may delegate the control and management of any school provided by them, with or without conditions or restrictions, to a body of managers appointed by them, consisting of not less than three persons.' Under this clause a large part of the local supervision of the schools in London is carried on. No better work can be undertaken by persons who care for children, and wish to add to the *esprit de corps* and happiness of their school life, and to take part in a most useful piece of local government. As a manager an almoner will find many occasions for timely and effective intervention.

XL.—RESTRICTIONS ON EMPLOYMENT.

In the recent Parliamentary and other inquiries in regard to 'Labour,' 'Sweating,' and the like, one suggestion has been frequently repeated, that it is desirable to enforce and sometimes, it is added, to extend the Factory Act. Moreover, as children are so often assistant wage-earners in a family, it may be well to mention some of the legal restrictions on child labour. Cases, too, may come to the knowledge of the almoner, in which there are infringements of the Act in regard also to women and young persons, and these he may think it right to report to the Inspector of Factories.

The employment of labour regulated by the Factory and Workshop Act 1878, refers to (1) Textile, (2) Non-textile factories, (3) Workshops, (4) Workshops employing no children or young persons, and (5) Domestic workshops.[1] *(margin: Factories and workshops to which the Factory Act applies.)*

The definitions of the three former terms are as follows:—

' The expression " textile factory " in this Act means—Any premises wherein or within the close or curtilage of which steam, water, or other mechanical power is used to move or work any machinery employed in preparing, manufacturing or finishing, or in any process incident to the manufacture of cotton, wool, hair, silk, flax, hemp, jute, tow, china, glass, cocoanut fibre, or other like material, either separately or mixed together, or mixed with any other material, or any fabric made thereof: *(margin: Textile factories.)*

' Provided that print works, bleaching and dyeing works, lace warehouses, paper mills, flax-scutch mills, rope works, and hat works, shall not be deemed to be textile factories.

' The expression " non-textile " factory in this Act means— *(margin: Non-textile factories.)*

' (1) Any works, warehouses, furnaces, mills, foundries or places named in Part I. of the Fourth Schedule to this Act. [*i.e.* Print works, bleaching and dyeing works, paper mills, flax-scutch mills, earthenware works, lucifer-match works, percussion-cap works, cartridge works, paper-staining works, fustian-cutting works, blast furnaces, copper mills, iron mills, foundries, metal and india-rubber works, glass works, tobacco factories, letter-press-printing works, book-binding works.]

' (2) Also any premises or places named in Part II. of the said Schedule, wherein or within the close, or curtilage, or precincts of which steam, water, or other mechanical power is used, in aid of the manufacturing process carried on there; [*i.e.* hat works, rope works, bakehouses, lace warehouses, ship-building yards, quarries, and pit banks.]

' (3) Also any premises wherein or within the close, or curtilage, or precincts of which any manual labour is exercised by way of trade, or for purposes of gain, in or incidental to the following purposes, or any of them; that is to say—

' (*a*) In or incidental to the making of any article, or of any part of any article; or

' (*b*) In or incidental to the altering, ornamenting, or finishing of any article; or

' (*c*) In or incidental to the adapting for sale of any article,

[1] *See* the Factory and Workshop Act 1878, with introduction, copious notes, and an elaborate index, by Alexander Redgrave, Esq., C.B., 1885. It is only possible in this 'Introduction' to refer to a few of the leading points of the Act. The reader should consult Mr. Redgrave's book as to further details. The Factory and Workshop Act 1891 (54 & 55 Vict., c. 75) amends and extends the Act of 1878.

and wherein or within the close, or curtilage, or precincts of which steam, water, or other mechanical power is used in aid of the manufacturing process carried on there.

'The expression "factory" in this Act means textile factory and non-textile factory or either of such description of factories.

Workshops. 'The expression "workshop" in this Act means—

'(1) Any premises or places named in Part II. of the Fourth Schedule [*see* above] to this Act, which are not a factory within the meaning of this Act.

'(2) Also any premises, room, or place, not being a factory within the meaning of this Act, in which premises, room, or place, or within the close, or curtilage, or precincts of which premises, any manual labour is exercised by way of trade or for purposes of gain, in or incidental to the following purposes ; that is to say –

'In or incidental to the making, altering, repairing, adapting, etc., of any article [as above], and to which, or over which premises, room, or place, the employer of the persons working therein has the right of access or control.'

Inspectors ; their powers; and prosecutions under the Factory Act. It would seem, then, that the whole length and breadth of manufacture is fairly covered by this Act. For the enforcement of the Act there is a Chief Inspector, Mr. R. E. Sprague Oram, and forty-five inspectors, of whom four are Superintending Inspectors and one is Superintending Inspector of Workshops. There are also twenty-three junior inspectors for the United Kingdom, besides two female inspectors and fifteen inspectors' assistants.

The south and south-east of England is under one Superintending Inspector, Mr. E. Gould (Home Office, S.W.), who has districts 31 to 39 under his charge. Of these, four are Metropolitan districts, each under the charge of one or more inspectors and junior inspectors. The Superintending Inspector of Workshops, Mr. J. B. Lakeman (Home Office, S.W.), is the Inspector of Workshops for the county of London, in which the registered workshops number 15,543. One of the female inspectors, Miss M. E Abraham, has her headquarters also at the Home Office.[1]

The inspector may 'enter, inspect and examine at all reasonable times, by day or night, a factory and a workshop and every part thereof when he has reasonable cause to believe that any person is employed therein, and to enter by day any place which he has reasonable cause to believe to be a factory or workshop.' If he has reasonable cause to apprehend obstruction, he may take a constable with him ; he may require the production of registers and other papers ; and 'he may examine either alone or in the presence of any other person, as he thinks fit, with respect to matters under this Act, any person whom he finds in a factory or workshop, or whom he has reasonable cause to believe to be or to have been employed within the preceding two months.' He may also enter 'any room or place actually used as a dwelling as well as for a factory or workshop.'[2]

---

[1] Report of the Chief Inspector of Factories and Workshops, year ending October, 1893.

[2] *Cf.* Factory and Workshop Act 1891, 54 & 55 Vict., c. 75, s. 25. 'A room' [not a dwelling, as in the Act of 1878] 'solely used for the purpose of sleeping therein shall not be deemed to form part of the factory or workshop for the purposes of this Act ' (s. 31).

The report of the Chief Inspector contains a list of the prosecutions under the Act during the previous twelvemonth. Some of the entries are suggestive, and will throw light on the regulations to be quoted in the next paragraph. We take these:—

Nature of offence.	Amount of penalty.			Amount of costs.		
	£	s.	d.	£	s.	d.
'Having employed a child for full time who produced no school qualifications . . .	2	0	0	0	3	0
'Having employed a young person, under the age of 16 years, before the hour of 5 A.M., to wit, at 4 A.M.	2	0	0	0	4	0
'Having neglected to affix an Abstract of the Acts in his factory	1	0	0	0	2	0
'Having neglected to keep a register of young persons in the prescribed form . . .	1	0	0	0	2	0
'Employing six young persons under the age of 16 years for periods varying from five weeks to 15 months, without having previously obtained certificates of fitness for employment from the surgeon, and after having been cautioned by Mr. Lakeman with reference to this matter upon a former visit	3	0	0	1	10	0
'Employing one woman and one young person (female) all night on 29 March, 1893' . .	2	10	0	0	4	0

One or two regulations may be noted in regard to (1) certificates of fitness for employment; and (2) employment, meal hours, and prohibitions of employment.

(1) *Certificate of Fitness.*—Persons under the age of 16 cannot be employed beyond seven or, if the certifying surgeon for the district resides more than three miles from the factory, beyond thirteen days, unless the 'occupier' of the factory (or employer) has obtained a certificate of fitness from the certifying surgeon of the district. The certificate includes a statement that the surgeon, by the production of a certificate of birth or other sufficient evidence, has satisfied himself as to the age of the person. If the inspector considers any such person incapacitated for working the full time allowed by law, he may require the employment of the child to be discontinued, unless the certifying surgeon personally examines the child and certifies to his ability.

(2) *Employment and Meal Hours, and Prohibition of Employment.*— Children (*i.e.* persons under 14 years of age) may not be employed under the age of 11. After that age they may be employed in morning and afternoon sets or on alternate days only. In the former case the hours are from 6 or 7 A.M. to 1 P.M. or dinner time; or 1 P.M. or dinner time to 6 or 7: in the latter case they may be employed as if they were 'young persons,' but not on two successive days or on the same day in the week in two successive weeks.[1]

[1] This statement refers to the employment of children in textile factories; the arrangements differ a little in the case of non-textile factories and workshops. For Saturdays there are special hours for young persons and children.

If overtime is to be worked in a factory or workshop under exceptional conditions, notice has to be sent to the inspector 'not later than eight o'clock in the evening on which the child, young person, or woman is employed.' (*Cf.* Act: 1891, s. 14.)

The parent of the child has to ' cause his child to attend some recognised efficient school,' on either the alternate days, or the alternate mornings or afternoons in which it is not at work. Due allowance is made for reasonable causes of absence as defined in the School Board paper quoted above. These regulations apply to all factories and workshops, excepting, of course, workshops at which no young persons or children are employed, and domestic workshops.

Each week the occupier of the factory or workshop receives a certificate of attendances from the teacher of the school attended by the child—to be produced to the inspector if required, within the next two months.

Every occupier has, within the limits allowed by the Act, to specify in a notice affixed in the factory or workshop, the period of employment, the times allowed for meals, and whether the children are employed on the system of morning and afternoon sets, or of alternate days.

Young persons and women. In the case of young persons and women, the period of employment, inclusive of meal hours, has to be either between 6 A.M. and 6 P.M., or between 7 A.M. and 7 P.M. By a 'young person' is meant ' a person of the age of 14 and under the age of 18 years.' 'Woman' means a woman of 18 years and upwards. A child between the ages of 13 and 14 who has obtained the certificate, or made the attendances required by the Code,[1] is considered a ' young person.' With some exceptions, a child, young person, or woman may not be employed on Sunday.

Workshops in which neither children nor young persons are employed.

Women in workshops. There remain two kinds of workshops not yet specially referred to, ' workshops' in which neither children nor young persons are employed, and ' domestic workshops.' In the former the period of employment for a woman begins at 6 and ends at 10, and on Saturday 6 to 4. For meals and absence from work during the period of employment is allowed a specified period of (except on Saturday) not less than one hour and a half; and on Saturday an hour. A workshop is not deemed to be a workshop of this type unless the occupier serves a notice on the inspector to that effect.

' Domestic workshops.' A ' domestic workshop ' is one ' where persons are employed at home, that is to say, in a private house, room or place, which, though used as a dwelling, is by reason of the work carried on there, a factory or workshop within the meaning of this Act, and in which neither steam, water, nor other mechanical power is used in aid of the

[1] See p. cix. as to children between 13 and 14 ; and s. 26 of the Factory and Workshop Act.

mannfacturing process carried on there, and in which the only persons employed are members of the same family dwelling there.' [1]

'Children can only be employed in domestic workshops in the morning and afternoon. They cannot be employed on the alternate day system. The restrictions upon labour, etc., do not apply to women employed in domestic workshops as defined by this section. . . . Domestic workshops are exempted from the sanitary regulations of the Act, from the fixing actual times for work and meals, and from affixing notices in the workrooms. . . . But they remain under the supervision of the local authority in respect to sanitary condition. They are also precluded from working overtime. The penalties for violation of the regulations of the Act by occupiers of the workshops are much less than is provided in other cases.' [2]

'An occupier of a factory or workshop shall not knowingly allow a woman to be employed therein within four weeks after she has given birth to a child.' [2]

(3) *Sanitary Provisions.*—As to factories: A factory has to be 'kept in a cleanly state and free from effluvia arising from any drain, water-closet, earth-closet, privy, urinal, or other nuisance.' It must not be so overcrowded as to be 'dangerous or injurious to the health of the persons employed therein,' and it must be so ventilated as to avoid such danger or injury. Factories have also to be periodically washed, lime-washed, and painted. [3]

In the case of sanitary defects in factories or workshops (whether children and young persons are employed in the latter or not) and laundries, the inspector under the Factory Acts gives notice to the local sanitary authority; and if that authority does not within a reasonable time take proceedings to 'remedy or punish the act, neglect, or default,' the inspector may do so, recovering expenses, if successful in his prosecution, from the sanitary authority. [4]

In the case of workshops (defined as above), the local sanitary authority has power to enter, inspect, take proceedings, etc., to ensure that they are periodically washed, lime-washed, and painted; and, if the occupier fails to comply with its notice, it may itself carry out the work and recover the cost from the occupier. [5]

In the case of London, the local sanitary authorities, on the certificate of a medical officer of health or sanitary inspector, have to enforce the lime-washing, cleansing, or purifying of factories not under the Factory and Workshop Act of 1878, and of workshops and workplaces. [6]

(4) *Dangerous Trades.*—The last annual report of the Chief Inspector contains the amended special rules recently adopted in

---

[1] Factory and Workshop Act, s. 16.
[2] Redgrave, p. 61, and Act of 1891, s. 21.
[3] Act 1878, modified by Act 1891, s. 5, 3 (1), etc.
[4] Act 1891, ss. 2, 3 (1).   [5] Act 1891, s. 4.
[6] The Public Health (London) Act 1891 (*see* p. clvi.).

regard to persons engaged in lead smelting, the working of blue lead, and the production of white lead, red and orange lead, yellow lead, and colours. Rules are published in regard to the conditions under which electric accumulator works, the enamelling of iron plates, and the tinning and enamelling of hollow wire are to be carried on. The almoner is very likely to come across persons engaged in these trades, especially that of manufacturing white lead. A note of some of the rules adopted in regard to this trade will serve as examples of the kind of safeguards that should be put in force :—

(1) Respirators, overall suits, and head-coverings have to be worn by the men and women who are engaged in certain specified parts of the manufacture; and for women shoes and stockings to be worn during work have also to be supplied.

(2) No female can be employed without a certificate of fitness from a medical man. No person can be re-employed after absence through illness without a certificate from a medical man. The doctor has to visit the factory weekly and has to examine each worker individually. Every case of illness has to be reported to the inspector of factories for the district and to the certifying surgeon.

(3) The employer has to provide dressing rooms, a dining room, lavatories, and a cloak room, in which the ordinary clothes of all workers have to be kept apart from their working clothes. Each man and woman has to take a bath at least once a week and to wash in the lavatory before bathing. A register is kept in which are entered the dates at which each worker commences and leaves employment, and the date when each worker takes a bath. Sanitary drinks have also to be provided—such as 'Sulphate of magnesia 2 oz., water 1 gallon; essence of lemon sufficient to flavour.'

XLI.—CHILDREN WHO ARE MORALLY NEGLECTED OR REFRACTORY.

For the morally neglected or refractory there are four classes of schools, the Industrial School, the Reformatory School, the Truant School, and the Day Industrial School. These we shall refer to in turn, noting at the outset one or two general considerations.

Difficulties in dealing with neglected children. Some of the cases upon which it is most difficult to decide are those in which parents do not fulfil their responsibilities to a child, and the choice appears to lie between removing from them a natural obligation, and thus allowing them to expend on their pleasures a larger part of the proceeds of their labour, or sacrificing the future life of the child to the indifference of his parents. The difficulties that surround the question may be indicated by two or three sentences from a recent Report of the Inspector of Reformatory and Industrial Schools :—

'The law gives full authority to magistrates to force the parent to contribute towards the child's maintenance in our schools, but the abject poverty of the class from which the children are usually drawn, and the difficulties under the Summary Jurisdiction Act of enforcing the collection, contribute to keep down the amount by which the Treasury benefits. . . . I cannot urge too strongly that the parent, whose neglect or bad example have been more to blame in most instances than the special depravity of his child, should be made to share in the punishment, and should not, by being too lightly taxed, be placed in a better position as regards the maintenance and education of his child than men who, equally poor, have been more attentive to their parental duties. The latter has out of his earnings to find food, clothing, and school pence for his children. The former (at the best at a small cost, more frequently for nothing) gets rid of all responsibility with regard to his child, who is better clothed, better fed, and as well educated, and when ready to be discharged from the school of detention finds employment provided for him by the school authorities. Under these circumstances we need not wonder if we find parents frequently driving their children into truancy, so as to qualify for an industrial school, rather than endeavouring to keep them out. For this the only remedy is to make such orders on the parent as will act as a deterrent, and to take care that these orders are rigorously enforced.

'Scarcely as many boys go to sea from our ships as we have a right to expect ; this is very much due to the action of the parents, who, careless to a culpable degree about their children when they are of an age to be a burden to them, evince an extraordinary affection for them and a great desire to have them at home when they arrive at an age when anything can be gained by their work. They, too often, use their influence to prevent their boys following up the life they have been educated for, and throw every obstacle in the way of their going to sea on discharge. Much would be gained if controlling powers could be given to managers of industrial training ships until the lad is seventeen or eighteen years of age.'

The Commissioners on Reformatory and Industrial Schools[1] draw special attention to the two points touched in this extract. They acknowledge very amply the good results of reformatory and industrial school training. 'The effect of the system of certified schools,' they say, ' has, on the whole, been very satisfactory. They are credited, we believe justly, with having broken up the gangs of young criminals in the larger towns ; with having put an end to the training of boys as professional thieves ; and with rescuing children fallen into crime from becoming habitual or hardened offenders. while they have undoubtedly had the effect of preventing large numbers of children from entering a career of crime.' They quote figures proving that since 1856, two years after the passing of the first English Reformatory Act, and one year before the first Industrial Schools Act, the number of the juvenile commitments to prison was 13,981; in 1866, 9,356 ; in 1876, 7,138 ; and in 1881, 5,483.

Further : ' Whereas in the quinquennial period of 1855-9 one sentence of penal servitude was inflicted to every 7,438 of the population, the proportion has steadily decreased, until in the year 1881 there was only one sentence to 17,028.' Yet some of their principal criticisms have regard to the abuse of the power of committing children to industrial schools. ' There is,' they say, ' ample testimony to the fact that this power has been largely abused, often from benevolent motives, sometimes because of the facilities afforded by the law to parents to get rid of the burden of their children's

[1] Reformatory and Industrial School Commission 1885.

Use and abuse of reformatory and industrial schools.

support and education by throwing it upon the industrial school system.' Mr. Duffus's evidence on this point is worth quoting :—

'Mr. Duffus, representing the Aberdeen Parochial Board, told us that they "are alarmed at the facility with which parents divest themselves of their children, and get them into these schools," not regarding this as any disgrace, but talking of the school as "a seminary that their children have been fortunate enough to get into." And indeed, on the evenings of the annual social meeting, they take their acquaintances there to point out with satisfaction their children. Mr. Duffus stated that parents regard the reformatory in a different light, and would struggle hard to prevent their children being sent to one, but they look upon the industrial school " just as a hospital (*i.e.* endowed school) for them"—although, from the feeling of the people of Scotland in regard to pauperism, they would "struggle long and hard before they would be subjected to taking relief from the poor rates."'

There were in Great Britain on December 31, 1893, 51 reformatory schools, which cost in that year £111,174, towards which parents paid only £4,635. The number under detention was 4,101 boys and 595 girls, a marked decrease as compared with former years. In industrial schools there were 19,960 boys, 4,511 girls; and the cost (including truant schools) was £406,882, of which the parents paid only £15,736. The increase in the number of inmates in industrial schools is marked. Ten years ago (1883) there were only 15,043, and 3,737 girls in them. There are 12 truant schools, to which 1,940 boys were admitted in 1893. Two are connected with the London School Board, one at Highbury, where on December 31, 1893, there were 186 children, and one at Upton House, where there were 141. A day industrial school will probably be established at an early date in London. Of these there are 22 in Great Britain. Their cost was £31,075, to which the parents contributed £3,089.

Proposed alternatives to the committal of children to Industrial and Reformatory Schools.

The Commissioners proposed checks—(1) by way of alternatives to committal, (2) by prolonged control over children, and (3) by a better system of enforcing payments from parents. As to (1), they write:—'For slight offences the only alternative to the reformatory or industrial school is a fine or imprisonment; and as the fine falls on the child, who is unable, while the parent is often unwilling, to pay it, this sentence frequently involves imprisonment. Thus the only option left to the magistrate is either to let the child go unpunished, or to commit it to an industrial school, a reformatory, or a prison. We agree with numerous witnesses in recommending that, in all cases of offences by children, the magistrate should have the following alternatives open to him in place of these often inappropriate forms of punishment; namely—

The power to order boys under 14 to be whipped;

Or to impose a fine (with imprisonment in default) on the parent ;

Or to take security from the parent for the good behaviour of the child.

There should also be power to compel the attendance of the

parent in court.' They suggest that boarding-out might be applied in cases of many of the children who are orphans or deserted and are now sent to industrial schools. They suggest also the repeal of the 16th section (*see* p. cxxiii.) of the Industrial Schools Act that refers to 'refractory children.'

With regard to the control of parents over children sent to reformatory and industrial schools, they said that—

Increase of age of control over children sent to Reformatory and Industrial Schools.

'There is abundance of evidence that the age of 16 is full of danger to boys, and still more, perhaps, to girls emancipated from the care of these institutions. At that age they are too apt to be dragged back into vice or crime by evil influences, frequently these of their own parents, to the destruction of the good work effected at great pains and expense. A parent who has allowed his child to fall into evil ways, and who has shown little or no parental interest in its welfare during the earlier years of its detention, and has, perhaps, evaded the duty of contributing to its support, will often awaken to a keen interest in it as the moment approaches when it will be free from restraint, and has attained an age at which its earnings will be an acceptable addition to the family resources. Such a parent has, in our opinion, forfeited any right to exert over the child an authority more properly belonging to the managers of the school which has been undoing the evil effects of parental neglect, and fulfilling the duties which the parent had failed to perform in the education and training of his child.'

Their recommendation on this head is:—

'The managers' control should continue for two years after expiration of sentence, provided that, in the case of reformatory school inmates who are then over 19, such control should cease at 21; and while the original detention should not be prolonged beyond the term of sentence, licenses should be renewable till the date when the control ceases, with a power of revocation not leading to a longer detention than may be necessary to give a fresh start.'

As to the recovery of payments, the Commissioners show that, taking the average cost per head at reformatories at 7s. 6d. to 8s. per week, or £19. 10s. or £20. 16s. a year, the parents' average share of the burden is about £1 a year, or five per cent. At industrial schools the cost per head is taken at 7s. to 7s. 6d. a week, or £18. 5s. or £19. 10s. a year, and the parents' average share of the burden (including the parochial board payments in Scotland) is a little more than £1, or five per cent.

Proposals for reform as to recovery of contributions from parents.

Since the Summary Jurisdiction Act 1879, 'parents' contributions and the costs of a complaint to a court for non-payment have been deemed to be "civil debts" recoverable under that Act, *i.e.* by means of distress warrants.' These are so harsh a method, that there is general disinclination on the part of magistrates to issue them; and 'where they have been unsuccessfully resorted to, the difficulty of proving that the defaulter has the means to pay is so great, that the power to imprison in such cases (section 35) is practically useless.' Sir James Ingham, the Chief Metropolitan Police Magistrate, said:—

'I should like to have a word to say about the unwillingness of the magis-

trates to send to an industrial school.   You know the sixth section of the
Summary Jurisdiction Act has, in effect, made the parents absolutely irresponsible.
For my own part, I have a very great objection to send a boy to an industrial
school, unless it is absolutely necessary, on account of the absolute irresponsibility
of the parent.   I should treat the parent most severely, and if I found that the
child was left running about the streets, in consequence of the gross negligence
or the immorality of the parent, I should strike at the parent boldly; I would
not even treat him as he was treated before this sixth section was passed.   I
should treat him with hard labour and great severity.   It seems to me a scan-
dalous thing that the wickeder the parent the greater relief he should get.
The wicked parents are absolutely relieved from the burden of maintaining their
children, and that burden is cast upon others.   That is a state of things which I
think ought not to be permitted for a moment, and I am quite sure that you
would find those magistrates who now object to sending children to an industrial
school, much more ready to obey the law, if they felt that the parents did not escape.'

On this head the Commission recommend that the Guardians
should be the payers and collectors of all sums due for the maintenance of children in these schools.   The details of the plan of
collection suggested by them need not here be mentioned.   The
reforms that they proposed have to a certain extent been carried
out, though Bills on the subject have been published in nearly
every session of Parliament since they reported.   An Act which
applies to Scotland only allows of committal by a magistrate
to a day industrial school instead of an industrial school.   The
Custody of Children Act 1891 limits the control of the parent
under certain circumstances, in the case of children brought up by
another person ('person' including any school or institution).   The
managers of an industrial school are now entrusted with a child's
supervision till the age of 18; and committals to reformatory
schools may extend to the age of 19.   (See pp. cxxiii., cxxv.)

It is clear from all this that the difficulty that is found in the
administration of the Poor Law reasserts itself in a very grave form
in connection with reformatory and industrial schools.   Parents
are unscrupulous and ready to secure any small advantage in the
battle of life.   Any provision of relief by the State must be in
part punitive or repellent, or it will be too readily accepted.   If
the State, with its legal powers of exacting payment, is unable
to cope with the difficulty of enforcing parental obligations,
charity, except so far as it can effect its purposes by persuasion and
insistence, is weaker still, and her interference in these cases is
often productive of evil without any redeeming feature.   Also,
while there is this vast State machinery for dealing with this
class of cases, charity, as in its co-operation with the Poor Law,
should leave to it its proper work, and should restrict itself to
the exceptional case, which it would be unjust to treat as one
of the mass, or which cannot be included in the terms of the
Acts.   Thus guarding itself, charity may find it well to help parents
whose children require for a short period special discipline or
training, by obtaining their admission to homes.   Many homes for
various classes are mentioned in the Register.

XLII. Certified Industrial Schools.

For whom certified industrial schools are intended.

These are schools in which 'industrial training is provided, and in which children are lodged, clothed, and fed, as well as taught.' Their rules have to be approved by the Secretary of State, and they are under the inspection of the Home Office. Reformatory schools (see p. cxxiv.) are for children between the ages of 10 and 16 who have been convicted of an offence punishable with penal servitude or imprisonment. Industrial schools are for children 'apparently' under 14, exposed to vice and crime. A child may not be detained in such a school beyond the age of 16, except with his own consent in writing; but, by the Act of 1891, every child sent to an industrial school after the passing of that Act must remain up to the age of 18 under the supervision of the managers of the school. In the Industrial Schools Act four classes are specifically mentioned.[1] (1) A child—

'Found begging or receiving alms (whether actually or under the pretext of selling or offering anything for sale), or being in any street or public place for the purpose of so begging or receiving alms :

'Found wandering, and not having any home or settled place of abode, or proper guardianship, or visible means of subsistence ;

'Found destitute, either being an orphan or having a surviving parent who is undergoing penal servitude or imprisonment ;

'Frequenting the company of reputed thieves.'

To these are added by the Industrial Schools Amendment Act of 1880 (43 & 44 Vict., c. 15, s. 1)—

'A child lodging, living, or residing with common or reputed prostitutes, or in a house resided in or frequented by prostitutes for the purposes of prostitution ;

'Or that frequents the company of prostitutes.'

Any person may bring before two justices or a magistrate any child, apparently under the age of 14 years, that comes under any of the above descriptions.

If the magistrate finds that the child does in fact come under one of these descriptions, and he thinks it expedient to deal with him under the Act, he may send him to a certified industrial school.

The other classes of children that may be dealt with under the Act are—

Child-offenders under 12 years of age.

(2) A child apparently under 12 years of age who is 'charged before two justices or a magistrate with an offence punishable by imprisonment or a less punishment, but has not been convicted in England of felony or in Scotland of theft.' The magistrate may order the child to be sent to an industrial school—'regard being had to his age and the circumstances of the case.'

[1] 29 & 30 Vict., c. 118.

Children
beyond
control or
'refractory.'
(3) A child apparently under the age of 14 brought before the magistrate by his parent, step-parent, or guardian, who represents that he is unable to control him and desires him to be sent to an industrial school. In this case the magistrate may deal with the child under the Act, if on inquiry he is satisfied that it is expedient to do so. (29 & 30 Vict., c. 118, s. 16.)

Children in
Poor Law
schools
under 14.
(4) A child apparently under the age of 14 maintained in a workhouse or pauper school, or in a district pauper school, who is refractory, or the child of parents either of whom has been convicted of a crime or an offence punishable with penal servitude or imprisonment. In this case, on the representation of the Board of Guardians or School Board of Management or Parochial Board, the magistrate may give a similar order, if he thinks it expedient. (29 & 30 Vict., c. 118, s. 17.)

Arrange-
ments for
sending
child, etc.
The order must (in England) be made by two or more justices in petty sessions, or a police or stipendiary magistrate, or the Lord Mayor or an alderman of the city of London.

Under other Acts also authorities may send children to industrial schools.

Thus (5) by the Prevention of Crime Act (34 & 35 Vict., c. 112, s. 14), any children of a woman convicted of crime, or against whom a previous conviction of a crime is proved, may be sent to an industrial school by a magistrate, under the Industrial Schools Act, if they are under 14 years of age, and under her control and care at the time of her conviction for the last of such crimes, and if they have no visible means of subsistence, or are without proper guardianship.

(6) Children may also be sent to industrial schools on non-attendance orders under the Education Acts.

'If the parent of any child above the age of five years, who is under the Elementary Education Act 1873[1] prohibited from being taken into full employment, habitually and without reasonable excuse neglects to provide efficient elementary instruction for his child; or if any child is found habitually wandering, or not under proper control, or in the company of rogues, vagabonds, disorderly persons, or reputed criminals, it shall be the duty of the local authority, after due warning to the parent of such child, to complain to a court of summary jurisdiction, and such court may, if satisfied of the truth of such complaint, order the child to attend some certified efficient school.' If the order is not complied with, and no 'reasonable excuse' is forthcoming (i.e. that the nearest school was more than two miles away, or that the absence was due to sickness or some unavoidable cause), the court may, if the parent fails to appear or fails to satisfy it, order a penalty not exceeding five shillings with costs ; but if the parent satisfies the court that he has

[1] 39 & 40 Vict., c. 79.

taken all reasonable efforts to enforce compliance with the order, it may, without inflicting a penalty, order the child to be sent to a certified industrial school. And upon a second or subsequent case of non-compliance the court may order the child to be sent to a day industrial school, or, if it appears to the court that there is no such school suitable for the child, then to a certified industrial school.

In regard generally to the selection of the industrial school, the order to be made by the magistrate, court, etc., the following additional notes may be of use:—

It is not necessary that the school to which the child is sent should be within the jurisdiction of the justices or magistrate that make the order. The order must specify the time for which the child is to be detained at the school; but it cannot extend beyond the time when the child reaches the age of 16. A school conducted in accordance with the child's religious persuasion, which is entered on the order, must be chosen. If such a school is not chosen, the 'parent, step-parent, guardian,' or if there be none of these, 'the god-parent or nearest adult relative,' may object, and upon proof being forthcoming in regard to the child's religious persuasion, the child may then be sent to another school. The application to the magistrate must, however, be made either before the child has been sent to a certified industrial school, or within thirty days of his arrival at such a school. The applicant must also show that the managers of the school he names are willing to receive the child. At the school the child has religious instruction from a minister of his own persuasion. Pending inquiry or the choice of a home, the magistrate may order that the child be detained for not more than seven days in the work-house of the Union where he was found or resident. The expense of conveyance to the school is defrayed by the police authorities. The Secretary of State may order the transfer of a child from one industrial school to another.

The managers of a school are now entrusted with the supervision of a child to the age of 18.[1] They may arrange that the child be lodged at the dwelling of his parent or of any trustworthy or respectable person, while they teach, train, clothe, and feed him as if he were in the school itself. If they do this, they must report it to the Secretary of State. After 18 months of the detention they may allow him to lodge with any trustworthy or respectable person to whom they give a license for this purpose. This license is renewed every three months. The license may also be revoked at any time and the child recalled to the school, where he may then be detained for another three months and again placed out on license, provided (1) that the managers think the recall necessary 'for the protection of the child'; (2) that notification is sent to the Secretary of State;

Placing out children sent to industrial schools on license.

[1] Industrial Schools Act Amendment Act, 57 & 58 Vict., c. 33, 1894.

(3) that they again place the child out as soon as possible, at latest within three months of the recall, and notify this to the Secretary of State. A child ' placed out on license ' may be apprenticed, though the period of detention may not have expired. To be apprenticed he must have conducted himself well during his absence from the school.

Discipline of children at industrial schools. The offences of a child punishable by law while he is liable to be detained at an industrial school, and whether he be lodging at the school or not, are these :—

(1) If, being apparently above 10 years of age, he wilfully neglects and wilfully refuses to conform to the rules of the school, he may on summary conviction be imprisoned for not less than 14 days and not more than three months, with or without hard labour ; and he may subsequently be sent to a certified reformatory school.

(2) If he escapes from school or neglects to attend thereat, he may be apprehended without warrant, brought before a magistrate, and sent, at the expense of the school managers, to be detained at the school until his time expires.

(3) Should the child convicted of this offence be apparently above 10 years of age, he may, instead of being sent back to school, be punished as above (1).

Parents' payments. For the custody and maintenance of children, grants are made from the Treasury. In the case of children sent on the application of their parents, step-parents, or guardians, the Government grant cannot exceed 2s. per head per week. The parents are liable, if of sufficient ability, to pay 5s. a week ; and if this sum is not paid, on the complaint of the Inspector of Industrial Schools, his agent or a constable acting on his directions, the magistrate may require its payment, or that of any less sum which he may think fit, to the inspector or his agent, for a specific time or until further order. When the amount of the payment ordered exceeds the amount paid in respect of any child by the Treasury, the balance is paid to the school managers.

XLIII.—Reformatory Schools.

Conditions of admission to reformatory schools. The conditions of admission to reformatory schools are these :— The offender must be, in the opinion of the magistrate before whom he is charged, less than 16 years of age. He must have been convicted of an offence punishable with penal servitude or imprisonment. He may then be sentenced to imprisonment for ten days or longer, and subsequently sent to a certified reformatory school for as many as five and not less than two years. Now, however, he can under certain circumstances be detained beyond the age of 15. If he appear to the court to be not less than 12 years of age, or is proved to have been previously convicted of an offence punishable with penal servitude or imprisonment, the court may, in addition to, or in lieu of, sentencing him according to law to any punishment, order that he be sent to a certified reformatory school, and be there detained for a period of not less than three and not more than five years, so, however, that the period is such as will, in the opinion of the court, expire at or before the time at which the offender will attain the age of 19 years. Also in regard to the ten days' imprisonment a change has been made. The court (without prejudice to any of its other powers) may direct that the offender be ' taken to a prison or to any other place, not being a prison, and the occupier of which is willing to receive him, and be detained therein for any time not exceeding seven days, or, in case of necessity, a period not exceeding fourteen days, or until an order is sooner made for his discharge or for his being sent to a reformatory school, or otherwise dealt with under this or any other Act.' [1]

A child of less than 10 years of age cannot be sent to a reformatory unless he has been previously charged with an offence punishable with penal servitude and imprisonment, or sentenced by a Judge of Assize or Court of General or Quarter Sessions. There are provisions in regard to reformatory schools similar to those in the Industrial Schools Act, relating to the religious persuasion of the child, placing him out on license, his apprenticeship, etc., etc.

XLIV.—The School Board Authorities and Industrial and Truant Schools. [2]

In cases of the habitual neglect of children, it is best probably to refer to the School Board authorities in the first instance. 'If,' says the Education Act of 1876 (39 & 40 Vict., c. 79, s. 11), 'either (1) the parent of any child above the age of 5 years who is under this Act (see p. cviii.) prohibited from being taken into full time employment, habitually and without reasonable excuse neglects to provide efficient elementary instruction for his child; or (2) any child is found habitually wandering, or not under proper control, or in the company of rogues, vagabonds, disorderly persons, or reputed criminals; it *shall* be the duty of the local authority, after due warning to the parent of such child, to complain to a court of summary jurisdiction.' The local authority is the School Board.

(margin: Powers of School Board in regard to neglected children.)

The magistrate may then make an attendance order, and if the child does not go to school the parent is fined 5s.; or if he has used all reasonable effort to get the child to school, the child may be sent to a day industrial school, or to a certified industrial school. If there is further non-compliance, there are further similar penalties. By the 13th section of the Act, if the School Board 'are informed

(margin: Attendance orders.)

[1] 56 & 57 Vict., c. 48, Reformatory Schools Act 1893.
[2] *See* The Elementary Education Acts, 1870 to 1880, by Hugh Owen; *see* especially pp. 251 *et seq.*

by any person of any child in their jurisdiction who is stated by that person to be *liable to be ordered* by a court under this Act to attend school, or to be sent under this Act or the Industrial Schools Act 1866, to an industrial school, it shall be the duty of the School Board 'to take proceedings under this Act or the Industrial Schools Act 1866, unless' the Board 'think it is inexpedient to take such proceedings.' If, then, any almoner or district visitor finds a child habitually away from school or neglected, he should write to the superintendent of the visitors in that division of the School Board.[1]

Industrial schools of the London School Board.

At Lady Day 1894 the School Board for London had under their management the following (*a*) industrial, and (*b*) truant schools, viz.: — (*a*) Brentwood (100 places), the ship 'Shaftesbury' (500 places) ; and (*b*) the Upton House Truant School (140 places), and the Highbury School, at Highbury Grove (200 places). They had also agreements with 35 voluntary industrial schools for boys, and 24 schools for girls ; and they have also use of accommodation at the Holme Court Truant School at Isleworth. At the above date there were, altogether, 1,308 children in industrial schools who had been sent at the instance of the Board, including 686 children (boys) at truant schools.

Short detention useful in truant cases.

There is one advantage in putting the School Board in motion, viz.: that, whereas by the Industrial Schools Act a child is not allowed to have a license to live outside the home until 18 months have expired, a child sent on the representation of the School Board can receive a license any time after one month's stay at the school.[2]

Truant Schools.

'It is desirable,' the Royal Commission on Reformatory and Industrial Schools reported, 'that children whose only offence has been truancy, either by their own fault or that of their parents, or who are unable by poverty to attend school, should be dealt with by terms of short duration in schools other than the reformatory and industrial schools.'

Truant schools have, it is said, been very successful where, as at Upton House, penal treatment, such as solitary confinement, is not resorted to, and where there is 'a shortened term of detention, amounting now, as a general rule, to about two months, or in a case of revocation of license, to about three months.' 'The essential features of the system seem to be a temporary deprivation of liberty, subjection to the regular hours and discipline of the establishment, daily schooling, plenty of drill, some industrial occupation, and very little play.' 'The results at the truant school at Upton House, to which, since November 6, 1878, all the worst cases of truancy

---

[1] *See* Industrial Schools, p. cxxi. ; and as to non-attendance of blind or deaf children, below, p. cxxxi.

[2] 39 & 40 Vict., c. 79, s. 15. *See* Elementary Education Acts, 1870 to 1880, by Sir Hugh Owen. p. 262.

among Protestant boys in the voluntary and Board schools of the Metropolis have been sent, are remarkable. Of 658 boys, 627 were licensed after an average absence from home of ten weeks and two days. In 252 cases the licenses were revoked, 204 boys were licensed a second time, and of these second licenses only 92 had to be revoked; 40 boys were licensed a third time, half of whom had their license revoked, and were transferred, with some of the other unsuccessful cases, making 92 in all, to ordinary industrial schools.

'In 1888 (to May) the percentage of possible attendance with these boys was 92·69.

'The subsequent attendances of the boys who had been truants have been considerably better than the average attendance of the other boys of the London Board schools.'

The question, indeed, is the same in schools of all kinds—the question of training *versus* beating. Mr. J. T. Kilner, of the Huddersfield Union, at a Poor Law Conference at Wakefield, in a paper on the treatment of workhouse children, put it as follows:—

Allow me to illustrate the treatment of an untractable child. His age is 8. He is a liar and a thief, has twice or three times attempted to set fire to his house, has been turned out of several schools, has killed a cat and a parrot, and is most incorrigible. Beating has no effect on him, his mother and his relatives are afraid of him, and no one can control him. Such is the problem placed before Mr. Steel at the Westminster Police Court by an anxious mother. Mr. Steel, however, could not answer the question, and merely suggested beating, beating, beating. Sir Edwin Chadwick says: 'I sent the statement of the case to Mr. Marshland, the superintendent of the district half-time school at Anerley, and asked for his observations on the case. I give his answer to it: "There needs no human Rarey to deal with a boy of this sort. Place him in better surroundings, give him no time to steal, ask him no questions for some time, and his habits of lying and stealing will die a natural death much quicker than by any amount of beating. Quite lately I had a boy with an inveterate habit of getting up in the night time and stealing from the clothes of his schoolfellows who slept in the same dormitory. I put him through an extra course of gymnastics before going to bed, and tired nature improved his moral nature. My remedy for a bad habit is to fill up boys' waking time with thoughts and actions of as pleasant a nature as possible, and with such a genial supervisor that the delight he takes in his new life leaves no room for his old life, and then send him to bed too tired to talk or do anything but go to sleep. Systematic and constant employment of time, made as pleasant as possible, never fails to alter and improve what are called incorrigible boys."'

Besides these schools, certified day industrial schools may be established if, owing to the circumstances of any class of the population in any school district, the Secretary of State thinks them desirable for the proper training and control of the children. In such schools industrial training, elementary education, and one or more meals a day, but not lodging, are provided.[1] A certified day industrial school will probably be established shortly in the Metropolis.

Children who may be sent to industrial schools under the Industrial Schools Act may, under 'an order of detention,' be sent,

Certified day industrial schools.

[1] Education Act, 39 & 40 Vict., c. 79, s. 16.

at the discretion of the court, to a certified day industrial school, if they are under 14 and found begging or receiving alms, etc. (*see* p. cxxi.); or frequenting the company of thieves; or, being under 12, are charged with an offence punishable by imprisonment or any less punishment, but not convicted in England or Ireland of felony, in Scotland of theft; or, being under 14 and under the care of a parent, are refractory (*see* p. cxxii.). They may also be sent under an attendance order, or if they have not complied with an attendance order.[1] The child is then detained daily during school hours, but he cannot be kept in this detention beyond three years or beyond the age of 14.

The certified day industrial schools are supported by grants from the School Board, by grants from the Treasury of not more than 1*s.* a head per week, and (where a child is sent by a court of summary jurisdiction, otherwise than by an attendance order) by contributions from the parents of not more than 2*s.* per week. If the parent is unable to pay, the Guardians, if satisfied of his inability to do so, 'shall give him sufficient relief to pay the said sum.' Children are also received into day industrial schools without any attendance order upon the request of a local authority, and of the parent of a child. The parent then pays not less than 1*s.* a week, and the Treasury may pay not more than 6*d.* per week for the child.

XLV.—THE BLIND, DEAF AND DUMB: THE POWERS OF THE GUARDIANS.

The Royal Commission on the condition of the Blind, the Deaf, and Dumb, etc. (1889), write:—

'The blind, deaf and dumb, and the educable class of imbeciles form a distinct group, which, if left uneducated, become not only a burden to themselves, but a weighty burden to the State. It is the interest of the State to educate them, so as to dry up as far as possible the minor streams which ultimately swell the great torrent of pauperism. Indigence is found to exist in the great majority of the cases of persons so afflicted.' An inquiry made by the Commission shows that out of 5,848 blind persons no less than 4,605 declare their inability to maintain themselves without charitable assistance, while only 959 state that they can so maintain themselves; 3,282 state that they earn nothing at all. 'It cannot be said that they are as a rule impoverished by any fault of their own; to deal with them, therefore, liberally in such matters as education or outdoor relief cannot be viewed as offering any reward to vice, folly, or improvidence. They are as distinct from the "pauper" in the ordinary sense as the "pauper" is distinct from the "criminal." . . . Their education is more expensive than that of ordinary children, and in many instances (especially in rural districts) necessitates the ex-

[1] Order in Council, art. 12; *see* Owen, pp. 264, 568.

pense of both education and maintenance. Fear has been expressed that, if their education were undertaken by the State, the effect might be to diminish that generous benevolence which has already done so much for them in this country. When it is remembered how much remains to be done for them, it is obvious that, even if such aid be given, there will still be room for the action of private benevolence, which experience shows to be often stimulated rather than discouraged by State aid when judiciously given.'

We take from the report the following note in regard to the prevention of blindness[1] :—

It is stated that 'a frequent cause of blindness is the inflamma- *The preven- tion of blindness.* tion of the eyes of new-born infants, which can be prevented, and, if taken in time, cured. It has been found by the Ophthalmological Society that 30 per cent. of the inmates of asylums (*i.e.* schools for the blind) are blinded from purulent ophthalmia in early life ; and about 7,000 persons in the United Kingdom have lost their sight from that cause.' Dr. Glascott states :—

'It has been distinctly proved in the large maternity and foundling hospitals of the Continent that the percentage of cases of purulent ophthalmia in the new-born can be materially diminished by simply cleansing the eyes of all children with clean water as soon as they are born. More recently the number of sufferers has been further diminished by the use of antiseptics, such as weak solutions of boracic or salicylic acid, a two-per-cent. solution of carbolic acid, however, giving the best results. As a further development of the preventive plan of treatment, the method of Crédé has been introduced. It has the merit of being extremely simple, and very efficient. It consists in washing the infant's eyes with pure water as soon as it is born, and then by means of a drop-tube instilling a single drop of two-per-cent. solution of nitrate of silver into the eyes. This simple method of prevention should be known to, and carried out by, every midwife in the country, and, what is more, parents should insist upon its being done.'

The provision made for the blind and deaf or deaf and dumb *Powers of Guardians, etc., as to the blind and deaf and dumb adults and children.* has recently been greatly extended.

1. The Guardians of the poor may give 'necessary relief' to the lame, impotent, old, blind, and such other among them being 'poor and unable to work.' All categories of afflicted persons come under this definition, if they are 'poor and unable to work,'[2] irrespective of age.

2. The Guardians may relieve a blind or deaf and dumb wife, and the relief thus given will not be considered as relief given to the husband. Thus the husband will not become a pauper, owing to his being (as he would be under the ordinary law) the legal recipient of such relief, and he would thus keep the Parliamentary and other franchises.[3] He is liable to pay for her if he has the

[1] The almoner will find the papers of the Society for the Prevention of Blindness of use.
[2] 43 Eliz., c. 2.
[3] 4 & 5 Will. IV., c. 76, s. 56. This refers also to children under 16 ; but these are now dealt with under the Elementary Education (Blind and Deaf Children) Act 1893, s. 10, with certain exceptions (*see* p. cxxxi.), and in these cases relief given to the child under 16 would not be considered relief given to the parent.

means, but the relief is not relief to him so as to make him removable. The words are :—

'And be it further enacted, that from and after the passing of this Act all relief given to or on account of the wife, or to or on account of any child or children under the age of 16, not being blind or deaf and dumb, shall be considered as given to the husband of such wife, or to the father of such child or children, as the case may be, and any relief given to or on account of any child or children under the age of 16 of any widow shall be considered as given to such widow.' Nothing in the Act is, however, to discharge relations responsible under 43 Eliz., c. 2, of that responsibility.

3. The legal responsibilities of parents towards children and children towards parents in regard to maintenance are, in the case of the blind and deaf and dumb, the same as those fixed by the law in other cases (see *ante*, p. l.).

4. By 30 & 31 Vict., c. 106, s. 21 (1867), 'the Guardians may provide for the reception, maintenance, and instruction of any adult pauper, being blind or deaf and dumb, in any hospital or institution established for the reception of persons suffering under such infirmities, and may pay the charges incurred in the conveyance of such pauper to and from the same, as well as those incurred in his maintenance, support, and instruction therein.'

5. Next, as to children, the Guardians (*see* p. xcii.) may, under 25 & 26 Vict., c. 43, ss. 1 & 10 (1862), send a child to any certified school—*i.e.* any institution for the instruction of the blind, deaf, dumb, lame, deformed, or idiotic, but not a certified reformatory school. But the child must be an orphan or deserted by his or her parents or surviving parent, or one whose parents or surviving parent shall consent to the sending of such child to the said school.

And by 45 & 46 Vict., c. 58, s. 13 (1882), the Guardians may 'pay the reasonable expenses incurred in the maintenance, clothing, and education of such child whilst in such school, to an amount not exceeding such rate of payment as may be sanctioned by the Local Government Board for pauper children sent to such school,' anything contained in the 25 & 26 Vict., c. 43, notwithstanding.

'The Local Government Board sanctions six shillings as the weekly sum to be paid for each child under the above provision.'[1]

The Guardians may also, by 31 & 32 Vict. (1868), c. 122, s. 42, 'with the approval of the Local Government Board, send any poor deaf and dumb or blind child to any school fitted for the reception of such child, *though such school shall not have been certified* under 25 & 26 Vict., c. 43.'

The Elementary Education (Blind and Deaf Children) Act 1893 (56 & 57 Vict., c. 42, s. 13), however, limits the field of the

---

[1] Glen's Archbold, p. 201.

Guardians in this department of work. From the 1st July, 1894, the Guardians have been able to place in schools only blind or deaf children who are (*a*) idiots or imbeciles; or (*b*) resident in the workhouse or in an institution to which they have been sent by a Board of Guardians from a workhouse; or (*c*) boarded-out by Guardians.

The responsibility of a parent towards the maintenance of a blind or deaf and dumb child relieved by the Guardians remains intact, though he does not by the receipt of such relief become, in the eye of the law, a pauper (*see* above s. 2, where the section from 4 & 5 Will. IV., c. 76, s. 56, is quoted).

6. The Guardians can also pay the fees in non-pauper cases in which a blind or deaf child is 'attending, or proposing to attend, a non-Board School where fees are charged,' between the ages of 7 and 16 in the case of a blind, and 5 and 16 in the case of a deaf child. Further, where the Guardians are giving outdoor relief to a parent, they must make it a condition that elementary education is provided for his blind or deaf child, and must give further relief, if necessary, with that object (see *ante*, p. cxi.).

7. By 42 & 43 Vict., c. 54, s. 10 (1879) (*see* p. cvi.), the Guardians have a large general power. They may 'subscribe towards any asylum or institution for blind persons, or for deaf and dumb persons,' if the Local Government Board be satisfied that the paupers under the Guardians have, or could have, assistance therein in case of necessity.

XLVI.—The Blind, Deaf and Dumb: the Provision made by the School Board.

Till the year 1893 the Guardians were the only authority that could pay for the maintenance of blind or deaf and dumb children in schools ; and they could deal alike with the children of parents who were or were not in receipt of Poor-Law relief. By the Act of 1893, for the better provision for the elementary education of blind and deaf children in England and Wales,[1] the powers of the educational authorities in dealing with these children are clearly defined, and their field of work divided from that of the Guardians :—

1. It is now obligatory on the parent of a blind or deaf[2] child, except in the case of a deaf child under seven years of age, to cause it to attend school. The blindness or deafness is not a 'reasonable excuse ' ' for neglecting to provide efficient elementary instruction for the child '; nor is the fact that there is no school which the child can attend, within two miles.

[1] 56 and 57 Vict., c. 42.

[2] 'Blind' means ' too blind to be able to read the ordinary school books used by children.' 'Deaf' means ' too deaf to be taught in a class of hearing children in an elementary school.'

2. On the other hand, the school authority must make 'efficient and suitable provision.' They may do this by establishing or acquiring and maintaining a school certified for the purpose by the Education Department; or they may contribute to such a school for the education of such children under conditions approved by the Education Department, and 'arrange for boarding-out any blind or deaf child in a home conveniently near to the certified school where the child is receiving elementary education.' 'The expression " school " includes any institution in which blind or deaf children are boarded or lodged as well as taught, and any establishment for boarding or lodging children taught in a certified school. If there is no School Board which may serve as school authority for the area for the purposes of this Act, the District Council for that area may be the authority.

3. The expenses which the school authority may incur include 'the expenses of and incidental to the attendance of the child at a school, and of and incidental to the maintenance and boarding-out of the child while so attending, and the expenses of conveying the child to or from the school.' 'Maintenance' includes the supply of clothing.

4. The parent is liable to contribute such weekly sum as may be agreed upon between him and the local authority. If they fail to agree, a court of summary jurisdiction may arbitrate; and 'any sum so agreed on or settled may, without prejudice to any other remedy, be recovered by the school authority summarily as a civil debt.'

5. The parent is deprived of no franchise, right, or privilege, nor is subject to any disability or disqualification, by reason of the education afforded to his child.

6. The period of compulsory education extends to the age of 16 in the case of blind and deaf children, and no such child is entitled to total or partial exemption from the obligation to attend school.

'In London the blind children usually attend the ordinary day-schools, and share, as far as possible, in the instruction there given; but they also, on specified days, receive special instruction at centres, of which there are 20. The attendance at these centres ranges from one to 19. The position and times of meeting of the different centres are frequently altered to meet the varying circumstances of the scholars. The average number on the roll for the year ended at Lady Day 1894 was 175, and the average attendance 134.' 'Blind children who have not passed the second standard, although over seven years of age, are admitted into the infants' departments.'

School Board for London: Report, 1893-94.

For the instruction of the deaf and dumb there are now 17 centres. The addresses of these will be found in the Register. The average attendance of children is 375. There is a superintendent, 35 women and 10 men, and 24 assistant instructors. The teaching is on the oral system. So far as it can be arranged no teacher has more than ten children under instruction. The arrangements for the attendance of children are similar to those for the blind. The superintendents of visitors send to the central office of the Board lists of the names and addresses of deaf children. They are then, if found suitable, sent to the nearest centre of instruction.

An almoner, on hearing of a blind or a deaf and dumb child who does not go to school, should communicate with the superintendent of the School Board visitors in the division, or with the clerk of the School Board, Victoria Embankment, E.C.

XLVII.—THE METROPOLITAN ASYLUMS BOARD.

As the charge of idiots and imbeciles and harmless lunatics is in London entrusted to the Metropolitan Asylums Board, who have also powers in regard to the supply of accommodation for the sick —the subject to which we pass next—it is convenient to state here the constitution of that Board. The Metropolitan Asylums Board was established under the Metropolitan Poor Act 1867. The Local Government Board were empowered to combine into districts ' unions or parishes, or unions and parishes ' in the Metropolis for the provision of asylums 'for the reception and relief of the sick, insane or infirm, or other class or classes of the poor chargeable in unions or parishes in the Metropolis.' Accordingly in May of that year the Board formed the Metropolis into one asylum district, under a board of management, since enlarged to 72 elective and nominated managers. The former (54) are elected by the Guardians; the latter (18) are appointed by the Local Government Board. Elected members may be chosen from among the Guardians themselves, or from among the ratepayers, but they must be rated to the poor-rate within the asylum district upon a net annual value of not less than £40.[1] Nominated members must be selected from among the 'justices of the peace for any county or place resident in the district,' or from among ' ratepayers assessed to the poor-rate therein on an annual rateable value of not less than £40,' or partly from the one and partly from the other.[1] They serve for three years. The Board has under its supervision the training ship ' Exmouth ' (see p. xcii.) ; four asylums—two for harmless lunatics, the asylums at Leavesden and Caterham, and two for imbeciles, the Darenth Adult Asylum and the Darenth Idiot School ; eight district hospitals, two hospital ships, and three ambulance stations, with three wharves and a river ambulance service. It has also had at Gore Farm a convalescent hospital for smallpox or fever patients (see p. cxli.).

[1] It would seem that the conditions as to rating, etc., attached to the appointment of members of the Metropolitan Asylums Board remain in force, although the qualifications of Guardians have been altered by the Local Government Act 1894.

XLVIII.—Lunatics. [1]

The almoner may in the course of his work have occasion to deal with cases of lunatic persons above the pauper class, for which he may desire to find accommodation. Or he may have to make arrangements for cases of pauper lunatics and cases of lunatics wandering at large.

The law regarding lunatics was consolidated by a Statute passed in 1890, and amended in 1891.

The supervision of institutions for lunatics, idiots, and imbeciles is in the hands of the Lunacy Commissioners. They consist of a chairman, one unpaid Commissioner, and six paid Commissioners, of whom three are legal and three medical. Each asylum is inspected annually by two or more Commissioners; each licensed house six times a year, or, if not within the immediate jurisdiction of the Commissioners, twice a year; each licensed hospital once a year. The Commissioners also visit lunatics, idiots, and imbeciles in workhouses, and unlicensed houses they visit once at least in the year. They publish an annual report.

The local control is vested in the case of (1) county and borough asylums, in the visiting committee of the county or town council. They have to visit once at least in every two months. (2) Licensed houses are visited by visitors consisting of three or more justices and one or more medical practitioners, appointed by the justices of the county or quarter sessions borough. They have to visit at least six times a year. (3) Further, institutions in which pauper lunatics are placed are visited by a medical practitioner appointed by the Poor Law Guardians of the union from which they have been sent, or by some of the Guardians themselves. Pauper lunatics who are not in an institution are visited by the medical officer of the union once a quarter. And lunatics who are in a workhouse must be visited once a quarter by the medical officer of the workhouse.

Lunatics may be detained in six ways, which entail expenditure from several different sources. They may be placed (1) in county or borough asylums. By the Local Government Act 1888, instead of grants in aid of local purposes being made from the Exchequer, it was arranged that the counties and 'county boroughs' should receive the proceeds of duties on local taxation licenses (licenses for the sale of intoxicating liquor on and off the premises, etc., etc.), and a grant from the proceeds of the probate duty. They were, in return, to make various payments to meet local needs. Amongst these are payments for the maintenance of pauper lunatics at the rate of 4s. a head per week, when the cost of such lunatics is equal to or exceeds that sum. The difference over and above the 4s. is made good from the rates. The counties and boroughs of a certain

[1] Lunacy Act 1890, 53 Vict. c. 5, and Amending Act 1891, 54 & 55 Vict., c. 65.

population are empowered to provide, maintain, enlarge, and visit asylums for pauper lunatics. Lunatics other than pauper lunatics can be received into county and borough asylums on payment, if there is room. (2) Lunatics may also be placed in licensed houses. These are institutions carried on for private profit. (3) Or they may be placed in registered hospitals. These are all, or almost all, supported by charitable endowments *plus* payments for patients. (4) They may be kept temporarily—under observation—in special wards of workhouses, or they may be retained in them, if harmless. (5) They may be placed under the care of relations; or (6) in un-licensed houses carried on for private profit. In this case not more than one patient can be received in the house.

Details on a few points may be of use to the almoner :—

1. *Non-Pauper Lunatics.*—Private patients may be found lunatic by judicial inquisition or by a petition for a reception order. In regard to the former it is only necessary to say that ' the Judge in Lunacy may, upon application by order, direct an inquisition whether a person is of unsound mind and incapable of managing himself and his affairs.' In certain circumstances the inquiry is made before a jury ; and in any case ' the inquisition shall be con-fined to the question whether or not the alleged lunatic is at the time of the inquisition of unsound mind and incapable of managing himself and his affairs ; and no evidence as to anything done or said by him, or as to his demeanour or state of mind at any time being more than two years before the inquisition, shall be receivable in proof of insanity, or on the trial of any traverse of an inquisition, unless the person executing the inquisition otherwise directs.' [1]

For the grant or refusal of reception orders, and other purposes, there is a ' judicial authority,' who may be a justice of the peace specially appointed for this purpose, year by year, by the justices of every county or quarter sessions, ' or a judge of county courts, or a magistrate, having respectively jurisdiction in the place where the lunatic is.'

'(1) The petition shall be presented, if possible, by the husband or wife, or by a relation of the alleged lunatic. If not so presented, it shall contain a statement of the reasons why the petition is not so presented, and of the connection of the petitioner with the alleged lunatic, and the circumstances under which he presents the petition. (2) No person shall present a petition unless he is at least 21 years of age, and has within 14 days before the presentation of the petition personally seen the alleged lunatic. (3) The petitioner shall in the petition undertake that he will personally, or by someone specially appointed by him, visit the patient once at least in every six months ; and the undertaking shall be recited in the order. (4) The petition shall be signed by the petitioner, and the statement of particulars by the person making the statement.'

The petition must be accompanied by a statement of parti-culars and by two medical certificates on separate sheets of paper --for all which forms required by the Act have to be used. The

[1] Part IV., Lunacy Act 1890.

judicial authority then makes further inquiry, if necessary, and grants or refuses the petition.

2. *Urgency Orders.*—

'In cases of urgency, where it is expedient, either for the welfare of a person (not a pauper) alleged to be a lunatic, or for the public safety, that the alleged lunatic should be forthwith placed under care and treatment, he may be received and detained in an institution for lunatics, or as a single patient, upon an urgency order, made (if possible) by the husband or wife, or by a relation of the alleged lunatic, accompanied by one medical certificate.'

No person shall sign an urgency order unless he is at least twenty-one years of age, and has within two days before the date of the order personally seen the alleged lunatic. The order remains in force seven days. For urgency orders the Act supplies forms.

No doubt in all these cases the almoner will obtain skilled advice for his guidance. The above notes only indicate the nature of the conditions which have to be fulfilled.

3. *Summary Reception Orders.*—

'Every constable, relieving officer, and overseer of a parish who has knowledge of any person within the district or parish of the constable, relieving officer, or overseer who is not a pauper and not wandering at large, is deemed to be a lunatic, and is not under proper care and control, or is cruelly treated or neglected by any relation or other person having the care or charge of him, shall within three days after obtaining such knowledge, give information thereof, upon oath, to a justice being a judicial authority under this Act.' The justice may in such case visit, or direct examination by two medical practitioners, and so proceed as in the case of a reception order, eventually, if desirable, sending the lunatic to some institution.

4. *Pauper Lunatics, and Lunatics wandering at large.*—The sections of the Act on these points we quote :—

'14. (1) Every medical officer of a union who has knowledge that a pauper resident within the district of the officer is or is deemed to be a lunatic and a proper person to be sent to an asylum, shall, within three days after obtaining such knowledge, give notice thereof in writing to the relieving officer of the district, or, if there is no such officer, to an overseer of the parish where the pauper resides.

'(2) Every relieving officer, and every overseer of a parish of which there is no relieving officer, who respectively have knowledge, either by notice from a medical officer or otherwise, that any pauper resident within the district or parish of the relieving officer or overseer is deemed to be a lunatic, shall, within three days after obtaining such knowledge, give notice thereof to a justice having jurisdiction in the place where the pauper resides.

'(3) A justice [not necessarily a "judicial authority" under the Act, but any justice], upon receiving such notice, shall by order require the relieving officer or overseer giving the notice to bring the alleged lunatic before him, or some other justice having jurisdiction in the place where the pauper resides, at such time and place, within three days from the time of the notice to the justice, as shall be appointed by the order.

'15. (1) Every constable and relieving officer and every overseer of a parish who has knowledge that any person (whether a pauper or not) wandering at large within the district or parish of the constable, relieving officer, or overseer is deemed to be a lunatic, shall immediately apprehend and take the alleged lunatic, or cause him to be apprehended and taken, before a justice.

'(2) Any justice, upon the information upon oath of any person that a person wandering at large within the limits of his jurisdiction is deemed to be a lunatic, may by order require a constable, relieving officer, or overseer of the district or parish where the alleged lunatic is, to apprehend him and bring him before the justice making the order, or any justice having jurisdiction where the alleged lunatic is.

'16. The justice before whom a pauper alleged to be a lunatic or an alleged lunatic wandering at large is brought under this Act shall call in a medical practitioner, and shall examine the alleged lunatic, and make such inquires as he thinks advisable, and if upon such examination or other proof the justice is satisfied in the first-mentioned case that the alleged lunatic is a lunatic and a proper person to be detained, and, in the secondly-mentioned case, that the alleged lunatic is a lunatic, and was wandering at large, and is a proper person to be detained, and if in each of the foregoing cases the medical practitioner who has been called in signs a medical certificate with regard to the lunatic, the justice may by order direct the lunatic to be received and detained in the institution for lunatics named in the order, and the relieving officer, overseer, or constable who brought the lunatic before the justice, or, in the case of a lunatic wandering at large, any constable who may by the justice be required to do so, shall forthwith convey the lunatic to such institution.

'17. Where, under this Act, notice has been given to, or an information upon oath laid before, a justice that a pauper resident within the limits of his jurisdiction is deemed to be a lunatic, and a proper person to be sent to an asylum, or that a person, whether a pauper or not, wandering at large within the limits aforesaid, is deemed to be a lunatic, such justice may examine the alleged lunatic at his own house or elsewhere, and may proceed in all respects as if the alleged lunatic had been brought before him.

'18. A justice shall not sign an order for the reception of a person as a pauper lunatic into an institution for lunatics, or workhouse, unless he is satisfied that the alleged pauper is either in receipt of relief, or in such circumstances as to require relief for his proper care. If it appears by the order that the justice is so satisfied, the lunatic shall be deemed to be a pauper chargeable to the union, county, or borough properly liable for his relief. A person who is visited by a medical officer of the union, at the expense of the union, is, for the purposes of this section, to be deemed to be in receipt of relief.

'19. (1) A justice making an order for the reception of a lunatic otherwise than upon petition, in this Act called a 'summary reception order,' may suspend the execution of the order for such period not exceeding fourteen days as he thinks fit, and in the meantime may give such directions or make such arrangements for the proper care and control of the lunatic as he considers proper.

'(2) If a medical practitioner who examines a lunatic as to whom a summary reception order has been made, certifies in writing that the lunatic is not in a fit state to be removed, the removal shall be suspended until the same or some other medical practitioner certifies in writing that the lunatic is fit to be removed, and every medical practitioner who has certified that the lunatic is not in a fit state to be removed shall, as soon as in his judgment the lunatic is in a fit state to be re-removed, be bound to certify accordingly.

'20. If a constable, relieving officer, or overseer is satisfied that it is necessary for the public safety, or the welfare of an alleged lunatic with regard to whom it is his duty to take any proceedings under this Act, that the alleged lunatic should, before any such proceedings can be taken, be placed under care and control, the constable, relieving officer, or overseer may remove the alleged lunatic to the workhouse of the union in which the alleged lunatic is, and the master of the workhouse shall, unless there is no proper accommodation in the workhouse for the alleged lunatic, receive and relieve, and detain the alleged lunatic therein, but no person shall be so detained for more than three days, and before the expiration of that time the constable, relieving officer, or overseer shall take such proceedings with regard to the alleged lunatic as are required by this Act.

'21. (1) In any case where a summary reception order might be made, any justice, if satisfied that it is expedient for the welfare of the lunatic, or for the public safety, that the lunatic should forthwith be placed under care and control, and if it appears to him that there is proper accommodation for the lunatic in the workhouse of the union in which the lunatic is, may make an order for taking the lunatic to and receiving him in that workhouse.

' (2) In any case where a summary reception order has been made, an order under this section may be made to provide for the detention of the lunatic until he can be removed.

' (3) An order under this section shall not authorise the detention of a lunatic in a workhouse for more than fourteen days, after which period such detention shall not be lawful, except in accordance with the provisions of this Act as to the detention of lunatics in workhouses.

' (4) An order under this section may be made by any justice having jurisdiction in the place where the lunatic is.

' 22. In the case of a lunatic as to whom a summary reception order may be made, nothing in this Act shall prevent a relation or friend from retaining or taking the lunatic under his own care, if a justice having jurisdiction to make the order, or the visitors of the asylum in which the lunatic is or is intended to be placed, shall be satisfied that proper care will be taken of the lunatic.'

As a rule, in cases of emergency it will be found best to apply to the relieving officer. The Chairman of a Board of Guardians may be authorised to act as a judicial authority under the following section of the amending Act[1] :—

' If, for the due administration of the Lunacy Acts, 1890 & 1891, in any union it appears to the Lord Chancellor desirable, he may, by writing under his hand, empower the Chairman of the Board of Guardians to sign orders for the reception of persons as pauper lunatics in institutions for lunatics, and every order so signed shall have effect as if made by a justice of the peace under the principal Act.'

A lunatic may not remain in a workhouse unless the medical officer certifies in writing that he is a proper person to be allowed to remain there, and that the accommodation is sufficient for his proper care and treatment. He may on this certificate be detained fourteen days. Lunatics not recovered may be discharged to a workhouse and there detained ; and chronic lunatics, not being dangerous, may be kept in a workhouse, by arrangement with an asylum and with the consent of the Local Government Board.

Reception orders may remain in force a year, and then two years, then three years, and so on up to five years, being renewed subject to report from the medical officer of the institution.[2]

XLIX.—IDIOTS AND IMBECILES.

' There is no clear line separating idiots and imbeciles ; it is merely a difference of degree, not of kind. Idiocy means a greater deficiency of intellect, and imbecility a lesser degree of such deficiency.' But the two, the idiot and the imbecile, are now definitely separated from the lunatic by the Idiots Act 1886, in which, ' if not inconsistent with the context, "idiots" or "imbeciles" do not include "lunatics," and "lunatic" does not mean or include "idiot" or "imbecile."' The formalities of the Lunacy Acts are set aside, and

[1] Lunacy Act 1891, 54 & 55 Vict., c. 65, s. 25.
[2] Act 1891, s. 7.

'a feeble-minded child can now be admitted into an institution to receive the benefits of its educational and industrial training upon a simple medical certificate that it is 'imbecile' and 'capable of receiving benefit from admission into an asylum.' The Lunacy Commissioners inspect all institutions, whether certified by the Local Government Board or not, which are registered or licensed under the Lunacy Acts for the reception of idiots and imbeciles, and they visit all workhouses where persons of unsound mind are detained. But there is no Government inspection of the education of educable imbeciles, nor general superintendence of the training and education of these classes.[1]

For the treatment also of cases of idiots and imbeciles the Guardians have large permissive powers. They may send 'idiotic persons' to certified schools by 25 & 26 Vict., c. 43 (*see* p. xcii.), and they may with the like consent send any idiotic, imbecile, or insane pauper who may lawfully be detained in a workhouse to the workhouse of any other union or parish, paying the cost of maintenance, etc.[2] They may, with the consent of the Local Government Board, send idiotic paupers to an asylum or establishment for the reception and relief of idiots maintained at the charge of the county rate or by public subscription.[3]

For imbecile children in the Metropolitan Poor Law area, the Metropolitan Asylums Board has an asylum at Darenth. And at the same place and under the same management is an asylum for adult imbeciles. Cases are admitted to these institutions through the Guardians. Application should be made to the relieving officer. The relief carries with it the disqualifications of pauperism. *Imbecile children.*

The Darenth Asylum is the only institution for idiots supported wholly by the rates In the rest of England there are seven Hospitals or Homes for Imbeciles registered under the Idiots Act; and there is some special provision for them in connection with one or two Lunatic Asylums, but the existing accommodation is altogether insufficient, and it is greatly to be desired that County Councils should have the power to establish for this class asylums similar to those at Darenth, to which both pauper and, on payment, non-pauper cases could be admitted.

L.—Feeble-minded, Epileptic, and Deformed.

Mention may here be made of some other classes of the afflicted, the feeble-minded, and deformed. The Royal Commission on the Blind, etc., inquired, at the request of the Royal Commission on the Elementary Education Acts, in regard to feeble-minded children.

[1] Report of the Royal Commission on the Blind, etc., p. xlv.; and Report of Special Committee of the Charity Organisation Society.
[2] The Idiots Act 1886, 49 & 50 Vict., c. 25, s. 15.
31 & 32 Vict., c. 122, s. 13.

Dr. Warner, a witness quoted by the Commission, thus states their condition :—

Need of separate classes and special education for feeble-minded children.

'Such cases as children who occasionally have slight epileptic fits, perhaps three or four in their lifetime, cases of slight chorea, cases of children who suffer from repeated sick-headaches, especially when attending schools, and who, upon that ground, are exempted; children whose nerve system is completely exhausted, and appears to have been so for months or years; cases of paralysis, of defective development from birth, cases of defective development of body, with slight defect of brain (I do not mean idiots); cases of nystagmus; cases of squinting; cases of myopia; cases of rickets, specially seen about the head with frequent co-incident nervous symptoms; and cases of diseased heart and lungs; these cases seem to require an exceptional method of education. Children who are suffering from any of the defects mentioned ought to be under exceptional methods of education. A large number of them are absent apparently without any certificate at all; only a few get certificates from me when they are my patients. (One hears at the East End of London they can buy them at 2d. apiece.) It is only in a few cases that patients of mine who, according to Act of Parliament, ought to be in attendance and who are absent, have asked me or any of my assistants for any certificate; and from inquiries that I have made in the schools, I believe that they are often absent without any certificate at all.'

Since this evidence was given a great advance has been made. Dr. Warner has, in connection with a committee of the British Medical Association, with a joint committee of members of that Association and members of the Charity Organisation Society, and subsequently, with a committee of the Sanitary Institute and Parkes' Museum, continued his investigations, so that now about 100,000 children have been examined. Public elementary schools and classes for feeble-minded children have been established, and (*see* Register) voluntary training homes for them have also been opened.[1]

A committee of the London School Board reported in 1891 in favour of the establishment of three schools of special instruction ' for those children who, by reason of physical or mental defects, cannot be properly taught in the ordinary standards or by ordinary methods.' Admission to these schools was to be arranged after examination of the child by a committee consisting of the Board inspector of the division, the Board's medical officer, and the local head teacher or superintendent of the school for special instruction. Not more than 30 children were to be under one teacher. The extended kindergarten system, with large liberty to the teachers to use the methods best adapted to the purpose, was suggested. On these lines one permanent school to accommodate 150 children, and eight temporary centres, have recently been opened.

Crippled, deformed, and invalid children.

Further reforms are desirable, that would give this class, as well as the lame, deformed, and epileptic, the same privileges as the blind or deaf in regard to elementary education either at day or boarding schools. (See *ante*, Section XLVI.)

With regard to adults, the 30 & 31 Vict., c. 106, s. 21 (1867),

[1] For recommendations on the whole subject, *see* the Report of the Special Committee of the Charity Organisation Society (1893), pp. 96 and 141.

which (*see* p. cxxx.) is now limited to the blind and the deaf and dumb, might be extended so as to enable the Guardians to provide for the reception, maintenance, and instruction of any pauper, adult, or young person of these classes above the legal age of education in any suitable hospital or institution.

For the provision of institutions for the care of epileptics, as the Register shows, an advance has also been made [1]; and possibly before very long groups of counties may each have their farm-colony and settlement for the education of children and the care and maintenance of adults who suffer from this disease.

The 'lame' and 'deformed' and crippled the Guardians have *Epileptics.* power (1) to send to a certified school under 25 & 26 Vict., c. 43, ss. 1 and 10; and (2) they may subscribe towards any asylum or institution for persons suffering from any permanent or natural infirmity under 42 & 43 Vict., c. 54, s. 10 (*see* p. cxxxi). Relief given by a Board of Guardians to a lame or deformed child does not carry with it the privileges of relief given to a blind or deaf-and-dumb child or wife under 4 & 5 Vict., c. 76; it is relief given to the parent or husband, and makes him a pauper.

LI.—Fever and Small-pox.

For the treatment of cases of fever and small-pox the Metropolitan Asylums Board has at its disposal the following institutions :—

Fever Hospitals.

1. Eastern Hospitals	Homerton, N.E.
2. North-Eastern Hospital	South Tottenham.
3. North-Western „	Haverstock Hill, N.W.
4. Western „	Fulham, S.W.
5. South-Western Hospitals	Stockwell, S.W.
6. Fountain Hospital	Tooting.
7. South-Eastern Hospital	Deptford, S.E.
8. Northern „	Winchmore Hill, N.

Small-pox Hospitals.

Hospital Ships 'Atlas' and 'Castalia'	Long Reach, Dartford, Kent.
Gore Farm Hospital, for convalescent small-pox or fever patients	Darenth, near Dartford, Kent.

Ambulance Stations.

Land Service—

Eastern Ambulance Station	Brooksby's Walk, Homerton, E.
South-Eastern „	Old Kent Road, S.E.
Western „	Seagrave Road, Fulham, S.W.

River Service—

The steamers 'Red Cross,' 'Maltese Cross,' and 'Albert Victor,' and the steam pinnace 'Swallow.'

Wharves and Piers.

North Wharf	Managers' Street, Blackwall, E.
South „	Trinity Street, Rotherhithe, S.E.
West „	Town Mead Road, near Wandsworth Bridge.

[1] *See* Report of Special Committee of the Charity Organisation Society on the Epileptic and Crippled, 1893.

Paupers must be such only as are infected or suffering from fever or small-pox.[1] They are admitted on an order, filled up and signed by a relieving officer, or master of a workhouse, accompanied by a certificate from the medical officer of the workhouse or district to which the person is chargeable, or by some registered medical practitioner, after due examination of the person proposed to be sent to the asylum.

Any person who presents himself at an asylum without the order and certificate may be admitted by the medical superintendent, if a refusal of admission would be attended with dangerous results; but a notice must be sent to the Guardians of the Union in which the patient last passed the night.

What to do in infectious cases.

The almoner, in any epidemic or in individual cases of cholera, small-pox, scarlet fever, diphtheria, &c., will find it useful to consult the papers of instructions issued, in the cheapest form, by the Local Government Board. Indeed he ought to make himself acquainted with them as a necessary part of his duties. If he finds a case, unknown to the medical officer of the Board of Guardians, he should at once inform him or the relieving officer.

To isolate the patient is all-important; and if he can be removed he will be sent in an ambulance provided by the Vestry or Metropolitan Asylums Board to one of their asylums. The notification of infectious diseases is compulsory.[2]

Cases which it may not appear desirable to send to these asylums, may be sent to the London Fever Hospital.

Non-pauper patients.

By the Poor Law Act 1889 (52 & 53 Vict., c. 56, s. 3), the Metropolitan Asylums Board may, subject to the regulations of the Local Government Board, admit to an asylum provided by them any person who is not a pauper, and is reasonably believed to be suffering from fever, or small-pox, or diphtheria. The expense thus incurred is to be 'paid by the Guardians of the Union from which the person is received, and those Guardians may recover the amount as a simple contract debt from the said person, or from any person liable by law to maintain him.' The expenses, so far as they are not recovered, are repayable to them out of the Metropolitan Common Poor Fund. The Local Government Board has authorised the Asylums Board to receive diphtheria patients.[3]

The Asylums Board, if they think fit, may allow their asylums for fever, small-pox, and diphtheria to be used for purposes of medical instruction.

---

[1] Local Government Board Orders, February 10, 1875, and June 7, 1887.

[2] With regard to compulsory notification of infectious diseases in London. See (6), p. clix.

[3] Local Government Board Order, October 11, 1889.

LII.—Metropolitan Common Poor Fund.[1]

While each union has to meet the cost of outdoor relief and other charges, a Metropolitan Common Fund, supported by contributions from all the metropolitan unions, in proportion to the annual rateable value of the property in them, has been established, under the Act of 1867 (sec. 69), to meet the expense of the Metropolitan Unions, under the following heads :—

(1) 'Maintenance of lunatics in asylums, registered hospitals and licensed houses, and of insane poor in asylums under this Act, except such expenses as are chargeable on the county rate.'

(2) 'Maintenance of patients in any asylum specially provided under this Act, for patients suffering from fever or small-pox.'

(3) 'All medicine and medical and surgical appliances supplied to the poor in receipt of relief by Guardians under this Act or any of the Poor Law Acts.' (See p. cxlvii.)

(4) Fees and other expenses of vaccination. (See p. cxlvii.)

(5) 'Maintenance of pauper children in district, separate, certificated, and licensed schools.'

(6) 'Relief of destitute persons certified by the auditor, and provision of temporary wards or other places of reception, approved by the Local Government Board, under the Metropolitan Houseless Poor Acts of 1864 and 1865.'

There are three other items of expenditure met by the Metropolitan Common Poor Fund—salaries and rations of all officers employed by the Guardians in and about the relief of the poor, of district school, asylum, and dispensary officers ; compensations to medical officers in case of determination or variation of contracts with them ; and births' and deaths' registration fees.

In 1869 an amending Act [2] was passed, by which, among other changes, it was arranged that 'the cost of the maintenance of pauper boys on board training ships; and the cost of the maintenance and instruction of orphan or deserted children placed out by the Guardians of any parish or union with the consent of the Local Government Board, should be repaid from the Metropolitan Common Poor Fund.'

In 1870, a further Act [3] placed the cost of indoor relief on this fund, on condition that the number of the paupers, together with the children under the age of 16 (if any), in any workhouse was not larger than the maximum fixed by the Local Government Board, and that the Guardians complied with the orders of the Board in regard to the alteration, enlargement, sanitation, furniture

---

[1] Metropolitan Poor Act (30 Vict., c. 6), s. 61.
[2] 32 & 33 Vict., c. 63, s. 21.
[3] 33 & 34 Vict., c. 18.

and fixtures, medical and surgical appliances, appointment of
officers, and classification of inmates. The rate of payment from
the Metropolitan Fund is 5*d*. a day per head for each indoor
pauper; and it was also arranged in 1870 that the cost of the
rations of indoor officers, according to a scale fixed by the Local
Government Board, should be repayable out of the fund.

In 1873 it was directed that the school fees paid by Guardians
for outdoor pauper children should be paid from the fund. (*See*
36 & 37 Vict., c. 86, s. 3, and 39 & 40 Vict., c. 79, s. 40, 1876.)

By the Poor Law Act of 1879, the expenses incurred by the
Metropolitan Asylums Board in providing ambulances, ambulance
stations, and horses, and in the conveyance of persons suffering
from any infectious disease, were charged to the fund; and by the
Poor Law Act of 1889, the Guardians are indemnified out of the
fund for expenses which are incurred on behalf of any non-pauper
patient admitted to the asylums of the Metropolitan Asylums
Board for small-pox, scarlet-fever, and diphtheria, but which they
cannot recover from the patient, or those liable to maintain him.

LIII.—THE SICK: CHARITABLE AND POOR LAW PROVISION.

The number of out-patients' letters that are circulated and the
ready admission of out-patients to hospitals frequently render
almoners altogether careless of the disposal of their 'letters.'
Sickness is treated as something apart from other distress. The
letter is at once given. Sometimes district visitors supply nourishing food—an invalid kitchen would appear to be a necessary adjunct
to a hospital—but in most instances the letter alone is given,
medicine is supplied, and nothing else is done. Yet as sickness is
so often the beginning of long-continued and sometimes irreme-
diable distress, it is then that everything should be done to make
cure rapid and certain. If a person is obtaining medical advice,
all that the doctor recommends—the 'feeding up' and the change
of air—should if possible be supplied. Often relief of other
kinds is required and may do much to facilitate recovery. Many of
the poor will not think of making any provision against the ordinary
sickness of life until they become ill. And the almoner, who has
helped a person through illness, should not think that his work is
done until he has induced him to join a friendly society or
provident dispensary.

One great cause of the carelessness of the poor to provide
against sickness is the out-patient system. Free medical relief
is ready everywhere to their hand. There is, it seems to them, no
reason why they should provide it at their own cost; and, since it is
so easily obtained, they come to claim it as a right. Well-established
hospitals make a fair show with their enormous number of out-
patient attendances. New hospitals start up and create a new

Misuse of hospital letters.

Out-patient departments and medical reform.

demand; and they advertise the large numbers who attend their
out-patient rooms, since monster statistics have an influence in
drawing contributions from those who do not analyse them and
seek their causes. If the number of new cases taken at out-
patient departments were limited, as is now done at St. Thomas'
Hospital, St. George's Hospital, and elsewhere, and the casualty
cases, which in these circumstances have a tendency to increase,
were kept within bounds, a beginning of reform would be made.
Cases required for purposes of medical study or teaching would be
kept in attendance with that object; others would receive advice
on their first visit only; and with the assistance of an almoner
or distributor of patients in the out-patients' department, working
in co-operation with local committees of the Charity Organisation Society and others, improper applications might be prevented, persons suitable for Poor Law treatment or for admission
to provident dispensaries might be referred to such institutions, and
cases in which other than medical relief is required might be otherwise aided. The power of almoners and subscribers to hospitals—
the possessors of the letters of admission—in promoting these and
other reforms is very great. The almoner should be a volunteer
canvasser on behalf of friendly societies and provident dispensaries.
In the Register will be found the medical benefits supplied by these
agencies.

In 1890, owing largely to the action of the Charity Organisation Society, a Select Committee of the House of Lords was
appointed to make inquiry into the management of hospitals and
dispensaries. One recommendation that they made will, it is hoped,
bear fruit—the establishment of a central body representing the
hospitals and dispensaries of the metropolis and some other institutions specially interested in the administration of medical relief.
Such a body might by degrees bring about a system of co-operation
between the hospitals and dispensaries, and, as opinion gradually
changed, might introduce improvements in methods of administration. The Select Committee suggested that the duties of the
Board should be of the following nature :— *A Central Hospital Board for London.*

'(1) It should receive annual reports, statements of accounts, and balance-
sheets from all hospitals and dispensaries, together with a return of the total
number of in-patients, out-patients, and casualty patients.

'(2) It should require that all accounts be audited by competent chartered
accountants.

'(3) It should arrange that all medical charities should be visited and reported
on periodically.

'(4) It should report from time to time, as occasion required, all proposals for
new hospitals.

'(5) It should publish an annual report, the principal heads of which might
be as follows :—

'(a) A complete statement as to the pecuniary position of each medical
charity.

'(*b*) A statement by a competent authority as to the existing sanitary condition and ventilation of each hospital, and as to arrangements concerted with the Metropolitan Fire Brigade.

'(*c*) An account of the number of beds in use, the number of beds unoccupied, and the reasons why they are unoccupied; the average daily number of occupied beds; details as to beds for which payment is made; and the number of resident medical staff, resident officers, nurses, and servants.

'(*d*) A statement as to the methods according to which each hospital deals with its out-patients and casualty patients, and the number of each.

'(*e*) Proposals for the removal of hospitals and dispensaries to places where further hospital or dispensary accommodation is required, and the proposals for the establishment of new hospitals, and all other matters relating to the treatment of the sick poor.

'(*f*) The nursing at hospitals, and the proceedings of nursing associations in the metropolis.

'(G) The proposed Board should early turn its attention to the possibility of so organising medical charity as to secure co-operation of hospitals and dispensaries with one another, and the co-operation of medical charity with general charity.'

Poor Law medical relief.

Overlapping and intercrossing the medical relief given by charitable institutions is a vast system of Poor Law medical relief. Since 1867 the Poor Law infirmaries have become hospitals; and in construction, medical treatment, and nursing they now take a high place. At the same time, the poor draw a distinction between the infirmary and the workhouse, and have no scruple in entering the former. To co-ordinate this system with the charitable medical system is one of the problems of medical reform in London at the present time, while in many instances admission obtained during illness is necessarily given with but little inquiry.

In the metropolis, under the Metropolitan Poor Act 1867, the Local Government Board have formed two districts. The Central London Sick Asylum District comprises Strand, Westminster, and St. Giles, and has an asylum at Cleveland Street, Fitzroy Square. It has also an asylum at Highgate, which is to be sold very shortly to the St. Pancras Union. The Poplar and Stepney Sick Asylum District, which includes these two Unions, has an asylum at Devons Road, Bromley. The managers of these asylums are partly elected by the Boards of Guardians concerned, partly nominated by the Local Government Board. They may[1] contract for the reception in the asylums of paupers chargeable to other unions; and if, under circumstances of urgency, they relieve at the asylums persons who are not paupers, all reasonable charges are, subject to restrictions of the Local Government Board, recoverable, and the relief given is deemed to be given by way of loan.[2] The asylums may be used for training nurses.

Guardians may subscribe to hospitals.

Guardians may,[3] with the consent of the Local Government Board, pay annual subscriptions towards the support and maintenance of any public hospital or infirmary for the reception of sick, diseased, disabled, or wounded persons, or of persons suffering from

---

[1] 39 & 40 Vict., c. 61, s. 22.   [2] 39 & 40 Vict., c. 61, s. 42.
[3] 14 & 15 Vict., c. 105, s. 4.

any permanent or natural infirmity. They may with similar consent also subscribe towards any association for providing nurses.[1]

Next with regard to the out-patient accommodation provided by the Poor Law (*see* local lists). The general medical Poor Law relief of a union is under the supervision of one or more medical officers. Unions are, if necessary, subdivided for medical purposes. In that case district medical officers are appointed to the several districts. But, except in the metropolis, no district is to contain more than fifteen thousand statute acres, or a population exceeding fifteen thousand persons. The medical officer has to attend and supply with medicine all the poor requiring medical attendance in his district, on an order from the Guardians or the relieving officer. If he attends a sick person without an order, he has to inform the relieving officer. *(margin: Poor Law outdoor medical relief.)*

In the Metropolis, under the Metropolitan Poor Act 1867, special provision is made for the establishment of Poor Law dispensaries in the several parishes and unions. The dispensaries are, if the Guardians so desire, placed under the management of dispensary visiting committees, of not less than five or more than nine, elected by the Guardians from their own body. Medical relief, as may be required, at the dispensary or at the patient's home, is given on an order to the district medical officer, signed by the relieving officer or the clerk to the Guardians. 'Urgent' is written on the order if the case is so considered. Drugs, medicines, and medical appliances are supplied. A dispenser and medical officer are in daily attendance, Sundays excepted. The cost of medicines, etc., and the salary of medical officers are charged to the Metropolitan Common Poor Fund, and if, on the requisition of the Local Government Board, they refuse or neglect to provide a dispensary, they forfeit the repayment from the fund. They may, with the consent of the Board, make arrangements for the treatment of paupers at some general hospital or dispensary.[2] *(margin: Poor Law dispensaries in the Metropolis.)*

LIV.—VACCINATION.

The influence of the almoner may be of lasting benefit in urging the poor to be vaccinated, especially at times when there is apprehension of small-pox.

Unions or parishes are divided into Vaccination Districts. These are in charge of Vaccination Officers, 'appointed to see to *(margin: Regulation as to vaccination.)*

[1] 42 & 43 Vict., c. 54. s. 10. 'The Guardians may, with the consent of the Local Government Board, subscribe towards any other asylum or institution,' besides those specified, which appears to the Guardians to be calculated to render useful aid in the administration of the relief of the poor. This would appear to include convalescent homes, &c. For the wording of this section of the Act, *see* p. cvii.

[2] 32 & 33 Vict., c. 6, s. 59. *See* Poor Law General Orders, Macmorran & Lushington, p. 514; and Metropolitan Dispensaries Order, April 22, 1871.

the execution of the Vaccination Acts, with a view of securing the vaccination of every child who is not unfit for it, or is susceptible of it.'[1] In each District is a Public Vaccinator, appointed and **Vaccination Stations.** paid by the Guardians; and there are Vaccination Stations, for the performance of vaccination. The Registrar of Births has, on or within seven days after the registration with him of the birth of a child not already vaccinated, to give notice to its parent or custodian, requiring the child to be vaccinated within three months; and he has to inform the parent of the place and hour at which the Public Vaccinator may be found. When the vaccination has taken place, and has after seven days been examined, a certificate, if the vaccination has been successful, is sent by the Public Vaccinator to the Vaccination Officer, and a duplicate is given to the parent. There are provisions for cases in which the child is unfit for vaccination, or where the operation is unsuccessful. If a medical practitioner, not the public vaccinator, performs the operation, the parent has to send to the Vaccination Officer, within 21 days of the operation, a signed certificate of successful vaccination, in accordance with a prescribed form. Neglect to vaccinate is punishable by a penalty of 20s.; and for neglect to transmit the certificate there is the same penalty.

The vaccination is free and not to be considered parochial relief.

The vaccination officer has to supply on demand a copy of the vaccination certificate at the cost of 6d. and 3d. for search. The Registrar receives 1d. in respect of every child whose birth he registers.

The Guardians may incur reasonable expenditure in circulating notices, making inquiries, or taking measures to prevent the spread of small-pox, and to promote vaccination upon any actual or expected outbreak of that disease in their Union.

If the vaccination officer informs a justice of the peace in writing that he has reason to believe that any child under 14 within the Union has not been successfully vaccinated, the parent may be summoned and required, unless the child is found to be unfit for or insusceptible to vaccination, on penalty of 20s. to have the operation performed.

LV.—THE VESTRIES AND DISTRICT BOARDS.

The Vestries and District Boards are the local sanitary authorities, and the Vestries are the rate collectors for the Metropolis. Their duties, their officers, and their constitution are interesting to the almoner chiefly owing to the fact of their being the sanitary authority. Questions are continually arising in which the intervention of the sanitary officers is desirable. Any person who has leisure and experience in executive work cannot do a greater service to the people at large than by becoming a member of the Vestry.

[1] Local Government Board Orders. Knight & Co., 1883. p. 800.

(1) The constitution of the Vestries and District Boards.— *Constitution of Vestries: elections, &c.* The Vestries and District Boards, together with the Metropolitan Board of Works, which has now been superseded by the London County Council (*see* p. cl.), were constituted on their present basis by the Metropolis Management Act 1855, and amending Acts. There are twenty-seven Vestries, the Woolwich Local Board, and twelve District Boards. By the Local Government Act 1894 the conditions of election and candidature of Vestries and the Woolwich Board are similar to those adopted in the case of Boards of Guardians [1] (*see* p. xxvi.). One-third of the Vestry retire annually, and their places are filled by newly-elected councillors. The District Boards consist of representatives of Vestries within their district.

Every Vestry and District Board has in June of every year to *Annual reports of Vestries and District Boards.* cause to be printed (1) an audited account in abstract and summary statement for the preceding year, (2) a report of their proceedings under the Metropolis Management Act, of works commenced, completed, or in progress, of proceedings in pursuance of any regulations of the general board of health for the time being in force, or otherwise for the removal of nuisances or the improvement of the sanitary condition of the parish or district; and (3) it has to append to its report a copy of every report of its medical officer. Copies of this 'account in abstract, statement and report,' together with a list of the names and addresses of officers, 'shall be delivered to any person applying for the same' for a sum not exceeding 2*d.*

The 'full statement and account' is to include the 'amount of all contracts entered into, and of all moneys received and expended' by the Vestry 'during the preceding year, all arrears of rates and other moneys then owing, all mortgages and other debts and liabilities.' [2]

(2) General Duties of the Vestries and District Boards.—To *Sanitary duties of Vestries and District Boards.* the Vestries and District Boards are entrusted the repair and cleansing of sewers, the paving, watering, cleansing, or improving of any parish or district, and 'all other duties, powers, and authorities in any wise relating to the regulation, government, or concerns of such parish.' [3] 'The affairs of the church,' and the legal relief of the poor are excepted. They are the authorities for establishing out of the poor rates public baths and washhouses, [4] and for providing burial grounds. They are the 'local authority' under the Metropolis Gas Act 1860 and the Public Libraries Act 1855. They appoint analysts under the Sale of Food and Drugs Act 1875.

---

[1] Ss. 23 and 30, and Local Government Order, November 3, 1894.
[2] Metropolis Management Act, 18 & 19 Vict., c. 130, ss. 192, 198.
[3] 18 & 19 Vict., c. 120, s. 90 (Metropolis Management Act 1855).
[4] 9 & 10 Vict., c. 74.

They are the rate collectors of the Metropolis. If the Guardians do not appoint a collector or assistant overseer to collect the poor rates,[1] the overseers on behalf of the Vestry collect them. Out of the poor rate the Guardians upon a precept from the Local Government Board pay into the hands of a 'receiver of the common poor fund' the amount of their contributions to the Metropolitan Common Poor Fund.[2] For the purposes of the Vestry the overseers make and levy a general rate, a sewers rate, and a lighting rate.[3] On the precepts of the Chief Commissioner of the Metropolitan Police, they levy the police rate; and on precepts from the School Board, the school rate. Till the Local Government Act of 1888, they used to raise the Metropolitan rate for the Metropolitan Board of Works. This, 'the county rate,' is now raised by the Guardians on the precepts of the London County Council.[4]

Among the sections of the Metropolis Local Management Act,[5] headed 'Annual Reports,' is the following :—

Duties of Vestries in regard to charitable trusts.

'Every such Vestry as aforesaid shall cause to be made out once at least in every year a list of the several freehold, copyhold, and leasehold estates, and of all charitable foundations and bequests, if any, belonging to the parish, and under the control of the Vestry, the list to contain a true and detailed account of the place where such estate or charitable foundation may be situate, or in what mode and security such bequest may be invested, specifying also the yearly rental of each, and the particular appropriation thereof, together with the names of the persons partaking of their benefit (except where such benefit shall be allotted to the poor of the parish generally), and to what amount in each case, and also stating the names and description of the persons in whom such estates are vested, and the names and description of the trustees for each charity, and such lists shall be open for the inspection of the ratepayers at the office of the Vestry Clerk at the same time with the accounts, when audited according to the provisions of this Act.' (*See* p. cxlix.).

LVI.—The London County Council.

By the Local Government Act of 1888, the Metropolis was formed into 'the administrative county of London.' The Metropolis is now 'the city of London and the parishes and places mentioned in Schedules A, B, and C to the Metropolis Management Act 1855, as amended by subsequent Acts.' The metropolitan area is thus the City of London and the area covered by the Metropolitan Board of Works, of which the Council is the successor. In charge of this area (with the exception of the City) is placed the London County Council, and to it were transferred the powers, duties, and liabilities of the Board of Works. The subordinate government of London, with its Guardians, vestries, and district boards, remained intact; but upon it was imposed, like

---

[1] Collectors of Poor Rates Order. Glen, p. 492.
[2] Metropolis Poor Act, 30 Vict., c. 6, s. 65.
[3] Metropolis Local Management Act, 18 & 19 Vict., c. 120, s. 161.
[4] *See* 'London Government,' Firth & Simpson, p. 82. The Commissioners of Sewers are the local authorities for the City of London.
[5] S. 199. Woolrych, p. 125.

a detached and separate thing, the County Council. It does not in any way represent the subordinate bodies, and is elected on a different franchise. Here it is not possible to do more than sketch in the merest outline its constitution and functions, and the following points only are referred to: the qualifications of electors and candidates; the duties of the Council, more particularly those inherited by it from the Metropolitan Board of Works and Quarter Sessions; and the contributions received by the Council from the Exchequer and distributed by it to Guardians and other local authorities.[1]

The Council consists of nineteen aldermen and one hundred and eighteen councillors. It holds office for three years. The electoral districts are the parliamentary boroughs. The franchise is that of the Local Government Register (see p. xxvii.).

The County Council: constitution: and franchise for its election.

'A person is not qualified to be a London County Councillor unless he is (1) registered and entitled to be registered as a London county elector, and also owns real property or personal property, or both, to the value of £1,000, or is rated to the poor rate in the county on the annual value of £30; or is (2) a peer owning property in the county; or is (3) registered as a parliamentary voter in respect of the ownership of property of whatever tenure situate in the county; or is (4) qualified to elect to the office of a London County Councillor and residing in the county. This provision (4) in effect dispenses with a property qualification. But if a person so qualified (4) ceases for six months to reside in the county, he ceases to be so qualified, and his office becomes vacant, unless he was at the time of his election, and continued to be qualified in some other manner. A person qualified as councillor for any one division of the county is qualified for every division. If, for example, he is registered in Chelsea, he can be elected in Camberwell.'[2]

Qualification of London County Councillor.

'The aldermen are elected by the elected members of the Council. Half retire at the close of the three years during which the elected members remain in office.'

Aldermen.

The London County Council inherited powers and duties chiefly from the Metropolitan Board of Works and from Quarter Sessions.

From the Metropolitan Board of Works it received charge of the general metropolitan drainage system. The main sewers are under its jurisdiction. It is entrusted with metropolitan improvements (such as the Thames Embankment), the supervision of building operations; it regulates the making of streets, their frontage

Duties of London County Council inherited from Metropolitan Board of Works.

---

[1] On the whole subject of the Local Government Act of 1888, *see* the 'County Councillor's Guide,' edited by Henry Hobhouse, M.P., and E. L. Fanshawe. W. Maxwell & Son, 8 Bell Yard, Temple Bar, 1888; and 'London Government,' by J. F. B. Firth, M.P., and E. R. Simpson. Knight & Co., 90 Fleet Street, E.C. 1888. Also Whale's 'Greater London.'

[2] Whale's 'Greater London,' p. 41. *Cf.* 'London Government,' p. 238.

and width, and the numbering of houses; and, with certain limitations, has power to make, widen, and improve streets and roads.
It has to keep the Thames free from obstructions, and to require
owners of land and premises on the riverside to do such works as
may prevent overflow into the metropolitan district. Under the
Loans Acts of the Metropolitan Board of Works, it has to borrow
money, create stock, and lend to local authorities in the Metropolis.
It has charge of the Thames bridges, the Thames tunnel, and the
Woolwich ferry. It appoints inspectors to test gas meters. It
is the metropolitan authority under the Metropolis Water Act 1871
which provides for a constant supply of water in the Metropolis,
outside the city of London. It is the local authority under the
Tramways Acts 1870, 1879, and is empowered to make bye-laws
to regulate the use of steam locomotives on highways under the
Highways and Locomotives Amendment Act 1878. As local
authority, it makes regulations under the Petroleum Act 1871 for
the conveyance and storage of petroleum and other similar oils;
and under the Explosives Act 1875 it grants licenses for the storage
of gunpowder. It enforces the Disused Burials Act 1884; and it
is the local authority under the Contagious Diseases (Animals) Acts
1878 and 1886. It is now also the authority under the Common
Lodging Houses Act 1851. It keeps the Register required under
the Infant Life Protection Act 1872 (*see* p. xcviii.). Under the
Metropolitan Fire Brigade Act 1865, it has the duty of extinguishing fires and protecting life and property in case of fire.

Open spaces.
To two of its inherited duties more special reference may be
made. Under the Metropolitan Commons Act 1866, it may present
a memorial to the Inclosure Commissioners with respect to any
common within the metropolitan area with a view to a scheme
for its management being prepared; and under the Metropolitan
Commons Act 1878, it can purchase and hold any saleable rights in
common with a view to the extinction of such rights and the
creation of an 'open space.'[1] Of its powers and duties under
various Dwellings Acts (*see* p. xcviii.).

Duties of
London
County
Council in-
herited from
Quarter
Sessions.
The legacy from Quarter Sessions to the Council includes,
amongst other duties, the following:—

'V. The licensing under any general Act of houses and other
places for music or for dancing, and the granting of licenses under
the Racecourses Licensing Act 1879.'

'VI. The provision, enlargement, maintenance, management,
and visitation of, and other dealings with asylums for pauper
lunatics' (*see* p. xxxiii.).

'VII. The establishment and maintenance of, and the contribution to, reformatory and industrial schools' (*see* p. cxxi.).

[1] *See* also the London Parks and Works Act 1887; the Garden in Towns
Protection Act 1863; the Metropolitan Open Spaces Act 1877; and the
Metropolitan Open Spaces Act 1881.

'XV. The registration of rules of scientific societies under 6 & 7 Vict., c. 36; the registration of charitable gifts under 52 Geo. III., c. 102 ; the certifying and recording of places of religious worship under 52 Geo. III., c. 155; the confirmation and the record of the rules of loan societies under 3 & 4 Vict., c. 110.'

To secure exemption from the rates scientific and loan societies must by the above-mentioned Acts deposit a copy of their rules with the County Council. The 52 Geo. III., c. 102, requires the registration of charitable trusts at Quarter Sessions.

One power of the Council derived from neither Metropolitan Board of Works nor Quarter Sessions must also be mentioned. The Council 'appoints medical officers of health, who shall not hold any other appointment, or engage in private practice without express written consent of the Council.' It is the central sanitary authority for the county. *Medical Officers of Health.*

By the (London) Equalisation of Rates Act 1894, the principle of the Metropolitan Common Poor Fund has been applied to sanitary expenditure. An Equalisation Fund is formed by the London County Council, equal to a rate of sixpence in the pound on the rateable value of London—according to the valuation lists— in each year. What each parish in London should *pay* to this fund is determined half-yearly by the London County Council, on the basis of a payment proportionate to the rateable value of each parish. What each sanitary district or parish should *receive* from this fund is determined by the size of the population of the district. If the sum payable by a parish on the sixpenny rate is *greater* than the sum receivable by it according to its relative population, the difference is used for grants *to* other parishes or sanitary districts ; but if the sum payable by it on the sixpenny rate is less than the sum receivable by it according to its relative population, a grant to make up the difference is received *from* the other parishes or sanitary districts. *Equalisation of rates for sanitary purposes.*

The grants have to be used by the sanitary authority in defraying expenses incurred 'under the Public Health (London) Act 1891, and, so far as not required for that purpose, those incurred in respect of lighting, and so far as not required for that purpose those incurred in respect of streets.'

A word or two in regard to the finances of the London County Council will show how—financially—the Council is brought into relation with the Poor Law Guardians and many other bodies. By the Local Government Act 1888, the Commissioners of Inland Revenue on behalf of the central government are to open a Local Taxation Account at the Bank of England, and they are to pay into it the duties on the local taxation licenses, which they are to continue to collect at least for the present. These are licenses [1] for the sale *The Exchequer contribution account; its receipts and expenditure.*

---

[1] Section 20 and Schedule I.

of intoxicating liquor on and off the premises; game licenses; licenses for dealers in beer, spirits, sweets, wine, tobacco, horses and plate; for dogs, killing game, guns, carriages, trade carts, locomotives, horses and mules, armorial bearings, and male servants; also for refreshment-house keepers, appraisers, auctioneers, hawkers, house agents, and pawnbrokers. Besides these the Commissioners are to pay into the Local Taxation Account a grant consisting of two-fifths of the Probate Duties. On their part the County Councils opened each of them an 'Exchequer Contribution Account,' and into th s are paid (1) the amount of the duties on local taxation licenses which have been collected in the county, and (2) from the two-fifths of the probate duties such a sum as the Local Government Board may certify to have been received by the county in grants from the Exchequer in the year ending March 25, 1888.

From these two sources the Council becomes possessed of means (I.) to make good certain grants to local authorities, which were before paid direct from the Exchequer; and (II.) to make certain extra grants to the Poor Law Guardians and Vestries or District Boards. As to the former, in London the Council has to pay [1] :—

I.

1. To the Guardians for every Poor Law Union or officer in any area wholly or partly in the county—

(a) Such sums as the Local Government Board from time to time certify to be due in substitution of the local grants towards the remuneration of teachers in Poor Law schools, and for payments to public vaccinators under section 5 of the Vaccination Act 1867; and

(b) Sums certified by the Local Government Board as payable in lieu of local grants for the remuneration of medical officers and the cost of drugs and medical appliances;.

(c) For the remuneration of registrars of births and deaths, a sum payable to Guardians in lieu of local grants, equal to the amount paid out of such grants for that purpose in the financial year to March 31, 1888; and

(d) Four shillings weekly for each pauper lunatic, if the net charge payable by the Guardians in such cases be four shillings or more; and

To County Fund for lunatics.

2. To the County Fund, for each pauper lunatic chargeable to the county and costing it that sum or more—four shillings;

3. Certain compensations to clerks of the peace and officers employed at Quarter Sessions (under 18 & 19 Vict., c. 126), and

Grant to police.

4. To the Receiver of the Metropolitan Police, the proportion of the cost of the police in the year ending March 31, 1888, which a

[1] Sections 24, 43, and 88. *See* for a short statement 'London Government,' p. xix.

Secretary of State certifies to have been contributed out of the Exchequer.

II.

Next, as to new grants to Poor Law Guardians and Vestries or District Boards. The Council in London has to pay—

5. To Vestries or District Boards one-half of the salary of each duly qualified medical officer hereafter to be appointed; and

To Vestries for medical officers hereafter appointed.

6. To Poor Law Guardians—

(a) The school fees paid for pauper children sent from a work-house to a public elementary school outside the workhouse; and

To Poor Law Guardians: School fees of workhouse children; indoor relief.

(b) For five financial years reckoned from the April 1, 1889 (or longer if Parliament so determine), fourpence per head for every indoor pauper. The number of the indoor paupers on whom the payment is to be made is to be the average number maintained by the Board of Guardians in the five years preceding March 25, 1888.

The term 'indoor pauper' includes all paupers maintained in the workhouse, district or separate school, separate infirmary, sick asylum, hospital for infectious diseases, institution for the deaf, dumb, blind, or idiots, certified school, boarded-out, and in asylums for imbeciles under the Metropolitan Asylums Board. 'Casual ward' paupers are excluded; and any number of paupers that there may be in a workhouse over and above the number prescribed by the Local Government Board.

These grants do not affect in any way grants made to Poor Law Guardians out of the Metropolitan Common Poor Fund.

This very brief sketch of the duties and powers of the London County Council, and of the qualifications of County Electors and County Councillors, will, it is hoped, be of service. It shows how great the powers of the Council are, and suggests how much greater they are likely to be. The work of the Council may seem to lie somewhat beyond the scope of the Introduction. In fact, however, it does not. The almoner can hardly be a capable almoner unless he be a good citizen, for he must find in the enforcement of the law not a little of the help which he needs in certain individual cases, and in a better general administration he will probably place his hopes of social progress, at least in certain departments of life. The County Council has not yet been brought into any systematic relation with the Vestries and District Boards. It in no way represents the local bodies that should co-operate with it, for instance, under the Public Health (London) and Housing of the Working Classes Acts; and it is likely that ere long further reforms will be made in the relation of the London County Council to the Corporation of the City, and possibly in that of the Vestries and District Boards to one another and to some central London

authority.   As these changes are made those who have sound
local knowledge of the civic administration and wants of any part
of London should try to influence public opinion in the right
direction.   But what is this 'right direction'?   Adam Smith says
that in Holland it was held to be 'unfashionable not to be a
man of business.   Necessity makes it usual for every man to be
so, and custom everywhere regulates fashion.'   Some kind of
compulsion akin to necessity, with custom and fashion in its train,
may yet make it usual in London for every man to be a citizen,
as well as a man of business.   Possibly then our local administration may be managed so as to draw out the interest of the
local ratepayer—or, perhaps, as we should now say, 'parochial
elector'—and require his active participation in local work.   This
to us seems the right direction.

LVII.—The London County Council and the Vestries and District Boards as Sanitary Authorities.

Sanitary,
Building,
and Housing
Acts.

Three groups of Acts are referred to in this section:—
I. The Sanitary Acts, consolidated in the Metropolis by the
Public Health Act 1891.   II. The London Building Act.   III. The
Dwellings Acts, consolidated in the Housing of the Working
Classes Act 1890.

I.—The Public Health (London) Act 1891.

A few of the main provisions of the Public Health (London)
Act 1891, 54 & 55 Vict., cap. 76, may be noted respecting
(1) nuisances; (2) offensive trades; (3) removal of refuse; (4)
unsound food; (5) provisions as to water supply; (6) notification
of infectious diseases; (7) cleansing and disinfecting of premises,
and the removal to hospital of infected persons without proper
lodging; and (8) ambulances.

(1) The first duty of the local sanitary authority is to 'cause to
be made from time to time inspection with a view to ascertain what
nuisances exist calling for abatement under the powers of the
Public Health Act,' and   .   .   .   'to secure the proper sanitary
condition of all premises within their district.'

The following nuisances may be abated summarily:—

'2.—(1) For the purposes of this Act,—
(a) Any premises in such a state as to be a nuisance or injurious or dangerous
to health;
'(b) Any pool, ditch, gutter, watercourse, cistern, water-closet, earth-closet,
privy, urinal, cesspool, drain, dung-pit, or ash-pit so foul or in such a
state as to be a nuisance or injurious or dangerous to health;
'(c) Any animal kept in such place or manner as to be a nuisance or injurious
or dangerous to health;
'(d) Any accumulation or deposit which is a nuisance or injurious or dangerous
to health;

'(e) Any house or part of a house so overcrowded as to be injurious or dangerous to the health of the inmates, whether or not members of the same family;

'(f) Any such absence from premises of water fittings as is a nuisance by virtue of section thirty-three of the Metropolis Water Act 1871, set out in the first schedule to this Act; and

'(g) Any factory, workshop, or workplace which is not a factory subject to the provisions of the Factory and Workshop Act 1878, relating to cleanliness, ventilation, and overcrowding, and

'(i) is not kept in a cleanly state and free from effluvia arising from any drain, privy, earth-closet, water-closet, urinal, or other nuisance, or

'(ii) is not ventilated in such a manner as to render harmless as far as practicable any gases, vapours, dust, or other impurities generated in the course of the work carried on therein that are a nuisance or injurious or dangerous to health, or

'(iii) is so overcrowded while work is carried on as to be injurious or dangerous to the health of those employed therein,

shall be nuisances liable to be dealt with summarily under this Act.

'(2) Provided that—

'(i) Any accumulation or deposit necessary for the effectual carrying on of any business or manufacture shall not be punishable as a nuisance under this section, if it is proved to the satisfaction of the court that the accumulation or deposit has not been kept longer than is necessary for the purposes of the business or manufacture, and that the best available means have been taken for preventing injury thereby to the public health; and

'(ii) In considering whether any dwelling-house or part of a dwelling-house which is used also as a factory, workshop, or workplace, or whether any factory, workshop, or workplace used also as a dwelling-house is a nuisance by reason of overcrowding, the court shall have regard to the circumstance of such other user.'

'Owner,' it may be added, in this Act means 'the person for the time being receiving the rack-rent of the premises in connection with which the word is used, whether on his own account or as agent or trustee for any other person, or who would so receive the same if such premises were let at a rack-rent.' Information¹ in regard to these nuisances may be given to the sanitary authority by any person, and 'it shall be the duty of every officer of that authority and of every relieving officer . . . to give that information.'

The power of entry of the sanitary authority is thus defined :—

'10. The sanitary authority shall have a right to enter from time to time any premises—

'(a) for the purpose of examining as to the existence thereon of any nuisance liable to be dealt with summarily under this Act, at any hour by day, or, in the case of a nuisance arising in respect of any business, then at any hour when that business is in progress or is usually carried on, and

'(b) where under this Act a nuisance has been ascertained to exist, or a nuisance order has been made, then at any such hour as aforesaid, until the nuisance is abated, or the works ordered to be done are completed, or the closing order is cancelled, as the case may be, and

'(c) where a nuisance order has not been complied with, or has been infringed, at all reasonable hours, including all hours during which business therein is in progress or is usually carried on, for the purpose of executing the order.'

(2) *Offensive Trades.*[1]—'Where any manufactory, building, or premises used for any trade, business, process or manufacture causing effluvia is certified to the sanitary authority by their medical officer of health, or by any two legally qualified medical practitioners, or by any ten inhabitants of the district of such authority, to be a nuisance, or injurious or dangerous to the health of any inhabitants of the district, such authority shall make a complaint to a petty sessions court.' A fine not exceeding fifty pounds may be levied, unless it is shown that the best practicable means for abating the nuisance have been adopted.

(3) *Removal of Refuse.*—The following clauses may be quoted :—

'29.—(1) It shall be the duty of every sanitary authority to keep the streets of their district, which are repairable by the inhabitants at large, including the footways, properly swept and cleansed so far as is reasonably practicable, and to collect and remove from the said streets, so far as is reasonably practicable, all street refuse.

'(2) If any such street in the district of any sanitary authority, including the footway, is not properly swept and cleansed, or the street refuse is not collected and removed from any such street, so far as is reasonably practicable, as required by this section, the sanitary authority shall be liable to a fine not exceeding twenty pounds.

'(3) So much of any Act as requires the occupier or owner of any premises in London to cause the footways and water-courses adjoining the premises to be swept and cleansed is hereby repealed.

'*Removal of house refuse.*

'30.—(1) It shall be the duty of every sanitary authority—

'(*a*) to secure the due removal at proper periods of house refuse from premises, and the due cleansing out and emptying at proper periods of ash-pits, and of earth-closets, privies, and cesspools (if any), in their districts, and the giving of sufficient notice of the times appointed for such removal, cleansing out, and emptying, and

'(*b*) where the house refuse is not removed from any premises in the district at the ordinary period, or any ash-pit, earth-closet, privy, or cesspool in or under any building in the district is not cleansed out or emptied at the ordinary period, and the occupier of the premises serves on the authority a written notice requiring the removal of such refuse, or the cleansing out and emptying of the ash-pit, earth-closet, privy, or cesspool, as the case may be, to comply with such notice within forty-eight hours after that service, exclusive of Sundays and public holidays.

'(2) If a sanitary authority fail without reasonable cause to comply with this section, they shall be liable to a fine not exceeding twenty pounds.

'(3) If any person in the employ of the sanitary authority, or of any contractor with the sanitary authority, demands from an occupier or his servant any fee or gratuity for removing any house refuse from any premises, he shall be liable to a fine not exceeding twenty shillings.

'*Sanitary authority to appoint scavengers.*

'(31) Every sanitary authority shall employ a sufficient number of scavengers, or contract with any scavengers, whether a company or individuals, for the execution of the duties of the sanitary authority under this Act with respect to the sweeping and cleansing of the several streets within their district, and the collection and removal of street refuse and house refuse, and the cleansing out and emptying of ash-pits, earth-closets, privies, and cesspools.'

---

[1] Sec. 21.

(4) *Unsound Food.*—Section 47 of the Act refers to this subject. The main clause of it is:—

'47.—(1) Any medical officer of health or sanitary inspector may at all reasonable times enter any premises and inspect and examine—

'(*a*) any animal intended for the food of man which is exposed for sale, or deposited in any place for the purpose of sale, or of preparation for sale, and

'(*b*) any article, whether solid or liquid, intended for the food of man, and sold or exposed for sale or deposited in any place for the purpose of sale or of preparation for sale,

the proof that the same was not exposed or deposited for any such purpose, or was not intended for the food of man, resting with the person charged ; and if any such animal or article appears to such medical officer or inspector to be diseased, or unsound, or unwholesome, or unfit for the food of man, he may seize and carry away the same himself or by an assistant, in order to have the same dealt with by a justice.'

Other clauses follow, stating the penalties for selling such food or exposing it for sale.

(5) *Provisions as to Water.*—A house without a proper and sufficient supply of water is now a nuisance. The sections on this point and on the cutting-off of the water supply are :—

'*Provisions as to house without proper water supply.*

'48.—(1) An occupied house without a proper and sufficient supply of water shall be a nuisance liable to be dealt with summarily under this Act, and, if it is a dwelling-house, shall be deemed unfit for human habitation.

'(2) A house which after the commencement of this Act is newly erected, or is pulled down to or below the ground floor and rebuilt, shall not be occupied as a dwelling-house until the sanitary authority have certified that it has a proper and sufficient supply of water, either from a water company or by some other means.

'(3) If the sanitary authority refuse such certificate, or fail to give it within one month after written request for the same from the owner of the house, the owner of the house may apply to a petty sessional court, and that court, after hearing or giving the sanitary authority an opportunity to be heard, may, if they think the certificate ought to have been granted, make an order authorising the occupation of the house ; but, unless such order is made, an owner who occupies, or permits to be occupied, the house as a dwelling-house without such certificate shall be liable to a fine not exceeding ten pounds, and to a fine not exceeding twenty shillings for every day during which it is so occupied until a proper and sufficient supply of water is provided ; but the imposition of such fine shall be without prejudice to any proceedings for obtaining a closing order.

'*Notice to sanitary authority of water supply being cut off.*

'49.—(1) Where a water company may lawfully cut off the water supply to any inhabited dwelling-house and cease to supply such dwelling-house with water for non payment of water rate or other cause, the company shall in every case, within twenty-four hours after exercising the said right, give notice thereof in writing to the sanitary authority of the district in which the house is situated.

'(2) Any company which neglects to comply with the foregoing provision shall be liable to a fine not exceeding ten pounds, and it shall be the duty of the sanitary authority to take proceedings against any company in default.

'(3) This section shall apply to every water company which is a trading company supplying water for profit.'

(6) *Notification of Infectious Disease.*—The following section (section 55) refers to this constantly-recurring question:—

'55.—(1) Where an inmate of any house within the district of a sanitary authority is suffering from an infectious disease to which this section applies, the following provisions shall have effect, that is to say:—

'(a) The head of the family to which such inmate (in this section referred to as the patient) belongs, and in his default the nearest relatives of the patient present in the house or being in attendance on the patient, and in default of such relatives, every person in charge of or in attendance on the patient, and in default of any such person the master of the house, shall, as soon as he becomes aware that the patient is suffering from an infectious disease to which this section applies, send notice thereof to the medical officer of health of the district :

'(b) Every medical practitioner attending on or called in to visit the patient shall forthwith, on becoming aware that the patient is suffering from an infectious disease to which this section applies, send to the medical officer of health of the district a certificate stating the full name and the age and sex of the patient, the full postal address of the house, and the infectious disease from which in the opinion of such medical practitioner the patient is suffering, and stating also whether the case occurs in the private practice of such practitioner or in his practice as a medical officer of any public body or institution, and where the certificate refers to the inmate of a hospital it shall specify the place from which and the date at which the inmate was brought to the hospital, and shall be sent to the medical officer of health of the district in which the said place is situate :

' Provided that, in the case of a hospital of the Metropolitan Asylum Managers, a notice or certificate need not be sent respecting any inmate with respect to whom a copy of the certificate has been previously forwarded by the medical officer of health of the district to the said managers.

'(2) Every person required by this section to send a notice or certificate, who fails forthwith to send the same, shall be liable to a fine not exceeding forty shillings: Provided that if a person is not required to send notice in the first instance, but only in default of some other person, he shall not be liable to any fine if he satisfies the court that he had reasonable cause to suppose that the notice had been duly sent.

'(3) The Local Government Board may prescribe forms for the purpose of certificates to be sent in pursuance of this section, and if such forms are so prescribed, they shall be used in all cases to which they apply. The sanitary authority shall gratuitously supply forms of certificate to any medical practitioner residing or practising in their district who applies for the same, and shall pay to every medical practitioner for each certificate duly sent by him in accordance with this section a fee of two shillings and sixpence if the case occurs in his private practice, and of one shilling if the case occurs in his practice as medical officer of any public body or institution.

'(4) Where a medical officer of health receives a certificate under this section relating to a patient within the Metropolitan Asylum district, he shall, within twelve hours after such receipt, send a copy thereof to the Metropolitan Asylum Managers, and to the head teacher of the school attended by the patient (if a child), or by any child who is an inmate of the same house as the patient. The Metropolitan Asylum Managers shall repay to the sanitary authority the fees paid by that authority in respect of the certificates whereof copies have been so sent to the managers. The managers shall send weekly to the county council, and to every medical officer of health, such return of the infectious diseases of which they receive certificates in pursuance of this section as the county council require.

'(5) Where in any district of a sanitary authority there are two or more medical officers of health of that authority, a certificate under this section shall be sent to such one of those officers as has charge of the area in which is the patient referred to in the certificate, or to such other of those officers as the sanitary authority may direct.

'(6) A notice or certificate to be sent to a medical officer in pursuance of this section may be sent to such officer at his office or residence.

'(7) This section shall apply to every building, vessel, tent, van, shed, or similar structure used for human habitation, in like manner as nearly as may be as if it were a house ; but nothing in this section shall extend to any house, building, vessel, tent, van, shed, or similar structure belonging to Her Majesty the Queen, or to any inmate thereof, nor to any vessel belonging to any foreign government.

'(8) In this section the expression "infectious disease to which this section applies" means any of the following diseases, namely, small-pox, cholera, diphtheria, membranous croup, erysipelas, the disease known as scarlatina or scarlet fever, and the fevers known by any of the following names, typhus, typhoid, enteric, relapsing, continued, or puerperal, and includes as respects any particular district any infectious disease to which this section has been applied by the sanitary authority of the district in manner provided by this Act.'

(7) *The Cleansing and Disinfecting of Premises.*—Section 60 is as follows :—

' 60.—(1) Where the medical officer of health of any sanitary authority or any other legally qualified medical practitioner, certifies that the cleansing and disinfecting of any house, or part thereof, and of any articles therein likely to retain infection, or the destruction of such articles, would tend to prevent or check any dangerous infectious disease, the sanitary authority shall serve notice on the master, or, where the house or part is unoccupied, on the owner, of such house or part, that the same and any such articles therein will be cleansed and disinfected or (as regards the articles) destroyed, by the sanitary authority, unless he informs the sanitary authority within twenty-four hours from the receipt of the notice that he will cleanse and disinfect the house or part and any such articles, or destroy such articles to the satisfaction of the medical officer of health, or of any other legally qualified medical practitioner, within a time fixed in the notice.

'(2) If either—

'(*a*) within twenty-four hours from the receipt of the notice, the person on whom the notice is served does not inform the sanitary authority as aforesaid, or

'(*b*) having so informed the sanitary authority, he fails to have the house or part thereof and any such articles disinfected or such articles destroyed as aforesaid within the time fixed in the notice, or

'(*c*) the master or owner without such notice gives his consent,

the house or part and articles shall be cleansed and disinfected or such articles destroyed by the officers and at the cost of the sanitary authority, under the superintendence of the medical officer of health.

'(3) For the purpose of carrying into effect this section the sanitary authority may enter by day on any premises.

' (4) The sanitary authority shall provide, free of charge, temporary shelter or house accommodation with any necessary attendants for the members of any family in which any dangerous infectious disease has appeared, who have been compelled to leave their dwellings for the purpose of enabling such dwellings to be disinfected by the sanitary authority.

'(5) When the sanitary authority have disinfected any house, part of a house, or article, under the provisions of this section, they shall compensate the master or owner of such house, or part of a house, or the owner of such article, for any unnecessary damage thereby caused to such house, part of a house, or article; and when the authority destroy any article under this section they shall compensate the owner thereof; and the amount of any such compensation shall be recoverable in a summary manner.'

(8) *Hospitals and Ambulances.*—Sections 75, 76, 77, and 78 are :—

' *Power of sanitary authority to provide hospitals.*

' 75.—(1) Any sanitary authority may provide for the use of the inhabitants of their district hospitals temporary or permanent, and for that purpose may—

' (*a*) themselves build such hospitals, or

' (*b*) contract for the use of any hospital or part of a hospital, or '(c) enter into any agreement with any person having the management of any hospital for the reception of the sick inhabitants of their district, on payment of such annual or other sum as may be agreed on.

'(2) Two or more sanitary authorities may combine in providing a common hospital.

'*Recovery of cost of maintenance of non-infectious patient in hospital.*

'76. Any expenses incurred by a sanitary authority in maintaining in a hospital (whether or not belonging to that authority) a patient who is not a pauper, and is not suffering from an infectious disease, shall be a simple contract debt due to the sanitary authority from that patient, or from any person liable by law to maintain him, but proceedings for its recovery shall not be commenced after the expiration of six months from the discharge of the patient, or if he dies in such hospital from the date of his death.

'*Power to provide temporary supply of medicine.*

'77. Any sanitary authority may, with the sanction of the Local Government Board, themselves provide, or contract with any person to provide, a temporary supply of medicine and medical assistance for the poorer inhabitants of their district.

'*Provision of conveyance for infected persons.*

'78. A sanitary authority may provide and maintain carriages suitable for the conveyance of persons suffering from any infectious disease, and pay the expense of conveying therein any person so suffering to a hospital or other place of destination.'

(9) *Bye-Laws for Lodging Houses.*—The sanitary authorities have power to make bye-laws as to lodging houses under the following section of the Act of 1891 :—

'94.—(1) Every sanitary authority shall make and enforce such bye-laws as are requisite for the following matters : (that is to say)

'(a) for fixing the number of persons who may occupy a house or part of a house which is let in lodgings or occupied by members of more than one family, and for the separation of the sexes in a house so let or occupied:

'(b) for the registration of houses so let or occupied :

'(c) for the inspection of such houses :

'(d) for enforcing drainage for such houses, and for promoting cleanliness and ventilation in such houses :

'(e) for the cleansing and lime-washing at stated times of the premises:

'(f) for the taking of precautions in case of any infectious disease.'

These bye-laws the almoner should obtain. They will probably differ in detail in different districts, but they will represent with fair accuracy what is the standard of sanitary requirement that should be aimed at in the dwellings of the poor. To the medical officer of the Vestry or the Inspector of Nuisances the almoner should complain in writing, if he comes across evils or defects which come within their jurisdiction. By endeavouring to have the law enforced in cases of overcrowding, defective sanitation, and other similar matters, the almoner can do acts of charity of untold value. The law is complete enough. But the poor are too often busy and too accustomed to bad sanitation to care about change.

Public Analysts.

Under the Sale of Food and Drugs Act (38 & 39 Vict., c. 63) 1875, Vestries and District Boards can appoint, subject to the approval of the Local Government Board, one or more persons possessing competent knowledge, skill and experience, as analysts of all articles of food and drugs sold within the district. Any medical officer of health, inspector of nuisances, or inspector of weights and measures, or any inspector of a market, or any police constable under the direction and at the cost of the local authority, may procure any sample of food or drugs. Any purchaser of an article of food or of a drug in any place where there is an analyst appointed under the Act may, on payment to him of a sum not exceeding ten shillings and sixpence, have the article analysed, and receive a certificate from the analyst.

' The person purchasing any article with the intention of submitting the same to analysis shall, after the purchase shall have been completed, forthwith notify to the seller, or his agent, selling the article his intention to have the same analysed by the public analyst, and shall offer to divide the article into three parts to be then and there separated, and each part to be marked and sealed, or fastened up in such manner as its nature will permit, and shall, if required to do so, proceed accordingly, and shall deliver one of the parts to the seller or his agent. He shall afterwards retain one of the said parts for future comparison, and submit the third part, if he deems it right to have the article analysed, to the analyst.'

II.—THE LONDON BUILDING ACT.

There is now a London Building Act.[1] It consolidates and amends the enactments relating to streets and buildings. It came into force on January 1, 1895. It provides for the formation and widening of streets, open spaces about buildings, and the height of buildings, construction, dangerous and neglected structures, dwelling houses on low-lying land, etc. It also (Sec. 164) gives to the London County Council the power to make bye-laws on many important points.

III.—THE DWELLINGS ACTS.

The Housing of the Working Classes Act[2] contains three parts which especially concern London. The first deals with unhealthy areas; the second, with unhealthy dwelling-houses; the third, with working-class lodging-houses.

Unhealthy areas are areas in which, owing to the badness of the houses, the narrowness, closeness, and bad arrangement of the streets, sanitary defects, etc., nothing short of an improvement scheme will prove an effectual remedy. An official representation respecting them may be made to the local authority (in the City, the Corporation, and outside the City, the County Council) by their medical officer of health, or any medical officer of health. 'A medical officer of health,' the fifth section says, 'shall make such representation wherever he sees cause to make the same; and if two or more justices of the peace, acting within the district for which he acts as medical officer of health, or twelve or more persons liable to be rated to the local rate complain to him of the unhealthiness of any area within such district, he must inspect and make an official representation on the facts of the case.' If an improvement scheme is carried out, accommodation has to be 'provided for at

[1] 57 & 58 Vict., c. ccxiii., 1894.　　　[2] 53 & 54 Vict., c. 70.

the least as many persons of the working-classes as may be displaced' in suitable dwellings, which, unless there are any special reasons to the contrary, shall be situate within the limits of the same area, or in the vicinity thereof, unless it is proved to the satisfaction of the confirming authority—a Secretary of State—that other equally convenient accommodation has been or will forthwith be provided, or where the local authority receives permission from the confirming authority freeing them from this obligation.

Unhealthy dwelling-houses—'buildings unfit for human habitation'—may 'be closed, and, if necessary, demolished by the order of the local authority' (in this part of the Act, the vestry or local board) :—

'30. It shall be the duty of the medical officer of health of every district to represent to the local authority of that district any dwelling-house which appears to him to be in a state so dangerous or injurious to health as to be unfit for human habitation.

'31.—(1) If in any district any four or more householders living in or near to any street complain in writing to the medical officer of health of that district that any dwelling-house in or near that street is in a condition so dangerous or injurious to health as to be unfit for human habitation, he shall forthwith inspect the same, and transmit to the local authority the said complaint, together with his opinion thereon, and, if he is of opinion that the dwelling-house is in the condition aforesaid, shall represent the same to the local authority, but the absence of any such complaint shall not excuse him from inspecting any dwelling-house and making a representation thereon to the local authority.

'(2) If within three months after receiving the said complaint and opinion or representation of the medical officer, the local authority, not being in the administrative county of London, or not being a rural sanitary authority in any other county, declines or neglects to take any proceedings to put this part of this Act in force, the householders who signed such complaint may petition the Local Government Board for an inquiry, and the said Board, after causing an inquiry to be held, may order the local authority to proceed under this part of this Act, and such order shall be binding on the local authority.

'32.—(1) It shall be the duty of every local authority to cause to be made from time to time inspection of their district, with a view to ascertain whether any dwelling-house therein is in a state so dangerous or injurious to health as to be unfit for human habitation, and if, on the representation of the medical officer, or of any officer of such authority, or information given, any dwelling-house appears to them to be in such state, to forthwith take proceedings against the owner or occupier for closing the dwelling-house under the enactments set out in the Third Schedule of this Act.'

Failing the closing order, the house may be demolished under the following section :—

'33.—(1) Where a closing order has been made in respect of any dwelling-house, and not been determined by a subsequent order, then the local authority, if of opinion that the dwelling-house has not been rendered fit for human habitation, and that the necessary steps are not being taken with all due diligence to render it so fit, and that the continuance of any building being or being part of the dwelling-house is dangerous or injurious to the health of the public or of the inhabitants of the neighbouring dwelling-houses, shall pass a resolution that it is expedient to order the demolition of the building.'

The third part of the Act deals with working-class lodging-houses, including 'separate houses or cottages for the working-classes, whether containing one or several tenements; and the purposes of this Act shall include the provision of such houses and cottages.' For this part in London outside the City the local authority is the London County Council. They are enabled by the Act to acquire land, or purchase existing lodging-houses, to 'erect any buildings suitable for lodging-houses for the working-classes, and convert any buildings into lodging-houses for the working-classes, and may alter, enlarge, repair, and improve the same respectively,' 'fit up,' 'furnish,' etc. They may make bye-laws for their regulation, and if the lodging-houses are found too expensive, they may sell them. But 'any person who, or whose wife or husband, at any time while such person is a tenant or occupier . . . receives any relief under the Acts relating to the relief of the poor other than relief granted on account only of accident or temporary illness, shall thereupon be disqualified for continuing to be such a tenant or occupier.'

Under this Act the London Council are building dwellings for the working-classes in various parts of London (*see* the Register).

There is thus placed in the hands of the municipality the amplest means of providing, for the labouring classes, lodging-houses at what rents and under what conditions they please. They may become the absolute managers of the houses, and they may, with the aid of the local rates, supplant private endeavour, wherever they may wish to do so. Impatient of slower processes, and even of 'enormous' improvements, they may apply this short and summary method of dealing with the ill-housed poor, trusting to their own sagacity to carry out, with good results to the community, that which others have failed to do.

Common Lodging-houses.—A common lodging-house is defined as that class of lodging-house in which persons of the poorer class are received for short periods, and, though strangers to one another [*i.e.*, not members of one family or household], are allowed to inhabit one common room. It does not include hotels, inns, public-houses, or lodgings let to the upper and middle classes.[1] It is a lodging-house often of a very rough description, at which the poor are housed for the night at about 4*d.* to 6*d.* a head. These houses have to be inspected on behalf of the County Council, now the local authority,[2] before they are opened as lodging-houses; and they are registered. The local authority may require a proper supply of water; the house has at all times to be open to inspection; the walls and ceilings have to be lime-washed in April and October of each year. The keeper of a common lodging-house, when a person in such house is ill of fever or any infectious or

Common lodging-houses: regulations regarding them.

[1] *See* page 96, Lumley's 'Public Health,' 3rd edition, by W. Patchett, Q.C., and A. Macmorran; and *cf.* 'A Treatise on Hygiene and Public Health,' edited by Stevenson and Murphy, Vol. III. Sanitary Law (p. 329).
[2] Common Lodging-houses Act 1851; and Local Government Order, May 7, 1894.

contagious disease, has to give immediate notice thereof to the local authority, and also to the Poor Law medical officer and the relieving officer of the union or parish in which the common lodging-house stands. Sick persons may be removed to a hospital; and in infectious cases, clothes or bedding disinfected or destroyed. Regulations for the management of these houses may be adopted by the local authority. The keeper of a common lodging-house in which beggars or vagrants are received must, if required by the Commissioners of Police, report every person who resorted to such house during the preceding day and night.

LVIII.—ENDOWED CHARITIES.

The creation of the Charity Commissioners was the first systematic attempt to provide for the proper administration of the charitable endowments in England and Wales, and to turn them to better uses. That race of poor persons known as 'gift-hunters' are sometimes kept in existence by the casual or periodic distribution of small charitable endowments, supplemented by similar voluntary alms. The injury that many of these endowments have done, and are doing, is incalculable. Their administration is frequently hampered by numerous restrictions, which necessitate a distribution to persons who comply with their conditions, rather than to persons who require their benefits. Their benefits are distributed rather with the object of satisfying the terms of a trust than in ways that would meet the special wants of an individual or a family in distress. They lose any remedial or really charitable element that they might possess if they were associated with the personal work and enthusiasm of the passing generation. And thus often they remain inadequate, inelastic, and official.

In 1870 Sir Arthur Hobhouse said [1] :—

'A charitable endowment or, in curt popular language, "a charity," has absolutely nothing to do with the virtue so called. It is simply a gift to be made to public uses, and to be governed for indefinite periods of time by the will of the giver. It need not be for the benefit of the poor; it need not be beneficial or wise; if not illegal or contrary to public policy—a source of objection which has been allowed an extremely narrow range—it is a good gift to "charity," and must take effect accordingly. Neither need it be made from any good motive.

'No ground of policy or expediency can be assigned for allowing [the founder] to dictate for ever, or for centuries, the mode in which his property shall be used. No human being, however wise and good, is able to foresee the special needs of society even for one or two generations. And yet our law says that anybody, although he may be a person whose opinion we should never think of taking in any subject whatever during his life, may compel us to take for all time property with almost any amount or kind of conditions not positively immoral. They may be foolish at the outset; change of circumstances may have made them useless or hurtful; still we must obey them. We do not allow such things to be done when the gift is to individuals or to families. An individual legatee, if he dislikes the condition, may decline the gift. . . . The consequences of so absurd a law are such as might be expected. The fruit is as the tree is. We have man-

[1] 'The Dead Hand.' Addresses on Endowments by Sir Arthur Hobhouse, Q.C.

aged our endowments according to the fortuitous views of myriads of testators, and the result is that until quite recently nearly the whole of these endowments were, and still a very large portion is, mismanaged so far as to produce in some cases no good, and in others positive injury to the persons affected by them.'

Under these circumstances, an almoner can hardly overlook almost the only machinery that exists for reforming these charities. It rests with the Charity Commissioners to remodel charitable trusts on wise principles; it rests with almoners and trustees throughout the country to give a new usefulness to these trusts by making them part and parcel of a well-organised system of individual charity. Possibly the clauses of the Local Government Act 1894, which place in the hands of the parish councils in rural districts a large share in the management of the parochial endowments, may, in the course of time, promote such a reform as this.

LIX.—Judicial Control over Endowments.[1]

A very ancient department of the jurisdiction of the Court of Chancery, now merged into the High Court of Justice, is that which relates to Charitable Trusts. The Court has jurisdiction to compel all trustees, and among them trustees of endowments, to perform the trusts reposed in them. In the case of endowments, which are for the benefit of the public and which never come to an end, the Court assumed a further jurisdiction, not existing in the case of ordinary trusts which are for the benefit of private individuals and which come to an end in, at least, the second generation after the donor's death. If the founder of an endowment failed to state his purpose with sufficient clearness, or if he omitted to prescribe the details requisite for carrying his purpose into effect, the Court could supply what was wanting. Again, if it was found that the particular objects contemplated by the founder did not exist, or if the details prescribed by him were found to be unworkable, the Court could remodel the arrangements But the Court has disclaimed the power of remodelling arrangements made by the founder merely because they are inconvenient or even pernicious to society.

The creation of a tribunal, with power to remodel pernicious or useless arrangements, is a cardinal point in dealing with endowments, is earnestly insisted on [2] by all who have studied the subject, and is sternly and successfully resisted by others. In order, therefore, that those who wish endowments to work well, instead of working in the way described in the preceding section, should have

The Court of Chancery and charitable endowments.

---

[1] *See*, for a most useful Memorandum on the origin and scope of the relations between the Charity Commissioners and the Trustees of Charities, Appendix A, 39th Report of the Charity Commissioners for England and Wales, 1882.

[2] *See* 'The Dead Hand,' quoted above ; also the Reports of the Charity Commissioners, etc.

a clear idea what is the defect in our law, it will be well to illustrate it by examples of circumstances in which the Court can and cannot alter the founder's arrangements. At a period of our history people were in the habit of devoting property to the ransom of Christians enslaved by the Mahometan powers. The time came when slaves of this kind ceased to exist. In these cases it has been held that the

Illustrations of difficulties in remodelling endowed charities.

Court can devote the property to some kindred purpose, *cy-près*, as the legal phrase goes. At the period of the Reformation, zeal for improved education led a great many persons to give property to maintain what were called grammar schools. What happened may be exemplified by the case of the Leeds School. In the year 1552 the founder had given property to pay a schoolmaster to teach in the Grammar School. In the early part of this century the people of Leeds wanted to learn other things than Greek and Latin, which alone were taught in the school. So the school became useless to them, and stood empty, or nearly so. The trustees and the Attorney-General proposed to introduce some modern subjects of learning. The schoolmaster resisted that. Lord Eldon decided in his favour. He held that it was not in the power of the Court to direct that anything but Greek and Latin should be taught in a grammar school. 'Other things might be very useful *to the people of Leeds*, but could not possibly be represented as useful *to that charity*.' In other words, an endowment in Leeds, for the people of Leeds, could not be made useful to them because the founder, nearly 300 years before, had contemplated, as the objects of his foundation, a schoolmaster to teach in a grammar school; and those objects, though useless and a scandal, were capable of existence.

The Leeds case is taken as a striking illustration, but is illustration only; not because it stood alone, for numbers of schools throughout the country were in a similar position, but because the requisite reform has been effected so far as regards educational endowments. As regards other endowments, they are still, with one exception, under the narrow law just set forth.

The Charity Commissioners and their powers.

Owing to its dilatory, cumbrous, and ruinously expensive procedure, the Court of Chancery was found totally inadequate as an administrator or supervisor of endowments. After attempts extending over fifty years, and during that time successfully resisted by the actual managers of endowments, a new machinery was created in the shape of the Charity Commissioners. They were established in 1853, and their jurisdiction was greatly enlarged in the years 1855 and 1860.[1]

(1) Inquiry and advice.

In the first place, they possess the important power of inquiring into the condition and administration of the great bulk of charitable endowments. They exercise this power through a staff of inspec-

---

[1] The principal Acts are 16 & 17 Vict., c. 137; 18 & 19 Vict., c. 124; 23 & 24 Vict., c. 136. Their office is at Gwydyr House, Whitehall.

tors, and they register annual accounts of the income and expenditure of the trustees. It is important to all persons interested in the working of an endowment to know that, by inquiring at the Charity Commission, they may obtain ample information—usually helpful advice—and if the case demands it, an inspection entirely free of cost. The broad light thus thrown on the working of endowments, and the constant communication of their trustees and others with a central authority, has already done more for their improvement than all the actions of the Court of Chancery for centuries.

In the second place, the Charity Commissioners have, by the establishment of official trustees, got a very simple machinery by which the safety of charity property is secured, and the expense of its devolution from one lot of trustees to another is saved, while the administration of the income by its managers is not interfered with. It is very important that this advantage to charity properties should be widely known. (2) Official trusteeship.

In the third place, the Charity Commissioners now exercise the old jurisdiction of the Court of Chancery in remodelling arrangements, or, as it is called, making new schemes. But the exercise of this power is subject to a very mischievous limitation. As regards small endowments, it may be exercised in every case; for the Commissioners may proceed to make a scheme on the application of the Attorney-General, or of any trustee of the endowment in question, or of any two inhabitants of the place it belongs to. But it is a curious instance of the dislike which the managers of these endowments have to reform, and of their great power in the legislature, that if the income of an endowment exceeds £50 a year, the Commissioners cannot make a scheme for it unless the trustees themselves ask to have one. For endowments worth £49 a year, it is a good thing that the Commissioners shall have jurisdiction upon being set in motion by agencies certain to be forthcoming if there is reasonable cause; but if an endowment has £51 a year, it may cry aloud for reform, the whole population of the place, a large minority of the trustees, and the Attorney-General may all be willing to ask for it, but the Commissioners cannot act unless a majority of the trustees themselves will ask to be reformed. Attempts have been made to remove this glaring absurdity, but hitherto the House of Lords have strenuously opposed the change. (3) Making new schemes. Limitations on Commissioners' powers.

The result of the establishment of the Charity Commission is that the old jurisdiction of the Court of Chancery, though it still exists in the High Court of Justice, is very rarely exercised. When the Commissioners find trustees obstinate, refusing to apply for a scheme, or when they find combative elements with which they cannot well deal, they call in the High Court. Otherwise the whole administration of charitable endowments is in their hands.

Educational endowments.

It has been before observed that educational endowments stand on a more favourable footing than others. A direct reform was effected by the Acts of 1869 and 1870, which not only established a tribunal (the Endowed Schools Commission) to remodel them without waiting till it pleased trustees or managers to be remodelled, but altered the law itself, so that the teaching and other arrangements might be brought into accordance with the needs of the public. It was also provided, in favour of education, that the trustees of useless endowments, notably dole-funds, might enable the Endowed Schools Commissioners to apply them to the purpose of education.[1]

The Endowed School Commissioners and the Charity Commissioners are now one and the same body. But it must always be borne in mind that with the important exception of endowed schools, and the small exception of the rarely used power given to trustees of useless endowments, there exist no legal means of remodelling an endowment because it has become useless and mischievous to society, or otherwise, than on the ground acted on by the Court of Chancery as above explained.[2]

The doctrine of cy-près.

The application of the doctrine of *cy-près* under the Charitable Trusts Acts has, however, been of late years greatly extended. In the comparatively recent case of the Campden Charities, Sir George Jessel, after referring to the entirely different circumstances of Kensington in Queen Elizabeth's time, when the trust was created, and to those of Kensington of the present day, said:—

'The next point is as regards the other half of Lady Campden's Charity, which is given in what is technically called doles. It is £5 per year to be distributed in two half-yearly payments to the poor alone, and in the church or porch thereof. That means 50s. each half-year, to be paid in money, in shillings and sixpences and half-crowns, to the poor people of the village who came to church. That is the practice in many parishes in England, and it is a practice which, I think, would be more honoured in the breach than in the observance. There is no doubt that it tends to demoralise the poor and benefit no one. With our present ideas on the subject, and our present experience, which has been gathered as the result of very careful inquiries by various committees and commissions on the state of the poor in England, we know that the extension of doles is simply the extension of mischief. That is a very great reason for not extending them if we can help it. . . . . That being so, and we being bound to administer the funds *cy-près*,

[1] The endowments which may be utilised (32 & 33 Vict., c. 56, s. 30) are those the income of which is wholly or partially applicable to doles in money or kind, marriage portions, redemption of prisoners and relatives, relief of poor prisoners in debt, loans, apprenticeship fees, advancement in life or any purposes which have failed altogether, or have become insignificant in comparison with the magnitude of an endowment for them—originally given to charitable uses in or before 1800.

[2] The preceding paragraphs of this section have been very kindly contributed.

what is the principal object which the testatrix had in view—as distinguished from the means by which she wished that object to be carried out? The principal object was to provide for the poor; and what poor? "For the relief of the most poor and needy that be of good life and conversation that should be inhabiting the parish of Kensington."[1] It was thus decided according to the scheme proposed by the Charity Commissioners to use the moiety of the endowment, referred to in the above quotation, in various sums to relieve cases of sudden sickness and other exceptional distress; for the aid of a hospital or dispensary, or nursing institution; for pensions; and for the encouragement of provident habits by contributions towards the payment of annuities. In the case of the City Parochial Charities the principle was adopted of resettlement of the non-ecclesiastical endowments with a view to the physical, moral, and social improvement of the poorer inhabitants, regardless of the special purposes for which the individual trusts were created.

Under a recent Act the Charity Commissioners are, in conjunction with the County Councils, conducting a most useful series of inquiries into the endowed charities of the several counties, and publishing a series of reports, which will form a New Digest of Endowed Charities, such as that issued by them some thirty years ago, but more complete.

The New Digest of Endowed Charities.

The following circular of the Charity Commission will show the reader what is required of trustees and others by the Charity Commission in the matter of accounts:—

'The Charitable Trusts Acts require that the trustees or persons acting in the administration of every charity shall, in books to be kept by them for the purpose, regularly enter or cause to be entered full and true accounts of all money received and paid respectively on account of such charity, and shall also on or before the 25th day of March in every year, or such other day as may be fixed for that purpose by the Board of Charity Commissioners, prepare and make out the following accounts in relation thereto (that is to say):

Circular relating to accounts. See 16 & 17 Vict., c. 137, s. 61; and 18 & 19 Vict., c. 124, s. 44.

' (1.) An account of the gross income arising from the endowment, or which ought to have arisen therefrom, during the year ending on the 31st day of December then last, or on such other day as may have been appointed for this purpose by the Board;

' (2.) An account of all balances in hand at the commencement of the year and of all moneys received during the same year on account of the charity;

' (3.) An account for the same period of all payments;

' (4.) An account of all moneys owing to or from the charity, so far as conveniently may be;

which accounts shall be certified under the hand of one or more of the trustees or administrators, and shall be audited by the auditor of the charity, if any; and that the said trustees or administrators shall, within fourteen days after the day appointed for making out such accounts, deliver or transmit a copy thereof to the Commissioners, at their office in London, and, in the case of parochial charities, shall deliver another copy thereof to the churchwarden or churchwardens of the parish or parishes with which the objects of such charities are

---

[1] See Charity Commission Acts, by R. E. Mitcheson (Stevens and Sons, 1887), and Tudor's Charitable Trusts, by L. S. Bristowe and W. J. Cook (Reeves & Turner, 1889).

identified, who shall present the same at the next general meeting of the Vestry of such parishes, and insert a copy thereof in the minutes of the vestry book; and that every such copy shall be open to the inspection of all persons at all seasonable hours, subject to such regulations as to the said Board may seem fit; and that any person may require a copy of every such account, or of any part thereof, on paying therefor after the rate of twopence for every seventy-two words or figures.'

The Local Government Board and endowed charities. The duties of the Vestries in regard to charitable trusts we have seen on p. cl. The Local Government Board have also authority in the matter, though it would seem probable that the enactment is practically obsolete.[1] They can require of all persons in whom are vested any property or funds belonging to any parish, and held in trust for or applicable to the relief of the poor, or which may be applied in diminution of the poor-rate, or of persons who are in the receipt of the rents, profits, or income of such property or funds, a true and detailed account in writing of the place where the estate is situated, or the manner in which the funds are invested. Details of the rents and profits and their appropriation have to be given, with all such other particulars relating thereto as the said Board may direct and require. This enactment applies only to endowed charities.

LX.—PAWNBROKERS.

Pawning and saving. Pawnbrokers are the bankers of the unthrifty. They give them advances on goods and household gear, and thus help them at a pinch. In a sense pawnbroking is a kind of inverse method of saving—taking credit for stock. And the poor will buy things, quite prepared to make capital out of them, in a time of need, and even estimating their prospective value for this purpose. 'The number and value of pawn-tickets' is a point on which information has to be obtained in most cases of distress, when the means at the disposal of the family for re-establishing themselves have to be reckoned up. Also a man who saves will often invest his money in furniture and other articles of worth. It is important, therefore, that the kind of goods pawned should be noted. If they be small articles they may be a sign of the constant unthrift of a needy family; if they be useful and of solid value they may indicate the break up of a good home.

Regulations regarding pawn-brokers. Pawnbrokers must have certificates from a magistrate.[2] They make the following charges : 'When a loan does not exceed 40s., $\frac{1}{2}d.$ per month on every 2s. or fraction of 2s. Half a month's charge if the pledge is redeemed within the first 14 days of any month except the first. When a loan exceeds 40s., $\frac{1}{2}d.$ per month, or part of a month, upon every 2s. 6d. or fraction of 2s. 6d. The charge for the pawn-ticket is $\frac{1}{2}d.$ if the loan is under 10s., 1d. if above. Upon loans between 40s. and £10, the parties may,

¹ 4 & 5 Will. IV., c. 67, s. 85.　　　² 35 & 36 Vict., c. 93.

if they please, make their own bargain, to be specified on a special ticket. All pledges are redeemable within 12 months and 7 days. A pledge for 10s. or under, if not so redeemed, is absolutely forfeited. Pledges over 10s. must be sold by public auction, and the pawnbroker is bound at any time within three years to account, upon demand, for the surplus.'[1]

LXI.—LOANS.

The assistance of those in distress by loan has been frequently advocated. The high percentage charged by loan societies makes them pitfalls for the distressed, rather than aids. The working man who has contracted such a loan is considered well-nigh doomed by his mates, so great are the chances against him. Yet a loan on good security without interest, or at a low interest, has helped many. The most convenient form for a loan is the following:—

Loans useful and useless.

PROMISSORY NOTE.[2]

I [or We jointly and severally] promise to pay to

being of the
the sum of
weekly instalments of
in every week, the first payment to be made on
In default of payment of any one instalment, the whole balance then remaining unpaid shall thereupon become due.

[or the Treasurer for the time
Charity Organisation Committee][3], or order,
, value received, by
shilling , payable on
.

[Date]

[Signed]

The stamps required are mentioned in the following note:—

By 33 & 34 Vict., c. 97, the duty on any bill of exchange of any kind whatsoever (except a bank note) and promissory note of any kind whatever (except a bank note), drawn, or expressed to be payable, or actually paid, or endorsed, or in any manner negotiated in the United Kingdom, is:—

Where the amount or value of the money for which the bill or note is drawn or made does not exceed £5 . . .	1d.
Exceeds £5 and does not exceed £10	2d.
„ £10 „ „ £25	3d.
„ £25 „ „ £50	6d.
„ £50 „ „ £75	9d.
„ £75 „ „ £100	1s.

By the same Act, section 54, every person who issues, indorses, transfers, negotiates, presents for payment, or pays any bill of exchange or promissory note liable to duty, and not being duly stamped, shall forfeit the sum of ten pounds ; and the person who takes or receives from any other person any such bill or note, not being duly stamped either in payment or as a security, or by purchase or otherwise, shall not be entitled to recover hereon, or to make the same available for any purpose whatever.

---

[1] 'The Justices' Note Book,' by W. K. Wigram, p. 344.
[2] This form of Promissory Note is to be given by a borrower alone, or by a borrower and surety or sureties.
[3] See 45 & 16 Vict., c. 61, s. 7.

Conditions of success in loans.

To make a loan effectual much care must usually be expended on the method of its repayment. There is not, as some would seem to think, any inherent virtue in a loan as against other forms of relief. It may be repaid and yet, like a gift, leave the borrower in as unsatisfactory a position as before. But a loan upon which sufficient care is spent may be as good a way as any of promoting thrift and foresight. In such a case the almoner should require that the instalment be paid weekly on a fixed day, and he should call for it himself, or arrange that it be called for on his behalf, or received at the rooms of some society. The former is the better plan, as it will thus be easier for him to induce the borrower to lay by in the savings bank the instalment, which, until his loan was repaid, he continued to pay to the lender. Of course this, like other good methods, requires constant personal care on the part of the almoner—a condition not always fulfilled.

Success in most instances depends rather on such care as this than on the actual form of the loan, for instance—with surety, or without surety, or as 'a returnable grant.' In special cases, at least, the loan with surety is advisable.

Loans with surety.

To ensure that the surety is satisfactory and that the payments are made punctually, the almoner would do well to employ such a society as the Charity Organisation Society. These loans must be treated as business, and on non-payment the borrower or his surety should, after due warning, be proceeded against by a summons to the County Court. It should be required that the instalment be paid on a fixed day in the week; and immediately on its non-payment a letter should be sent to the borrower. Subsequently if the payment is not made, he should be visited at once. The surety should be as nearly as possible in the same rank of life as the borrower. The borrower is then reluctant to let the security pay on his behalf. A surety in a better position in life than the borrower is inclined to think it a grievance if he has to make good his obligation. Loans, of course, should not be granted except in cases where there is a thoroughly reasonable prospect of repayment. Sometimes what may be termed a returnable grant may be a substitute, especially where there is a possibility rather than a prospect of repayment; and where care has been taken, these have been usually repaid as promptly and fully as loans. In such a case the applicant may be told that he is expected to pay: when the character of applicants has been ascertained by inquiry, it is often found that they readily make good this obligation. Sometimes part of the assistance may be by way of loan.

A typical loan case of the right character may be mentioned :—

A coppersmith of 30, who had been ill for five weeks, was referred to us by the relieving officer, who had granted relief for the first time. The man had three children under six, and was soon expecting another, and was getting 12s. a week from his trade society. His character from his employers was good, but he had dissipated his money in the past. The relatives were induced to do what they could; an allowance was begun. The Church gave 1s. 6d. a week; the club excused the man his arrears and exempted him from payment for a quarter; clothes were granted; a relative was induced to take one girl; the man was sent to a convalescent home; the wife was helped after her confinement, and sent by a mothers' meeting to the country. On the man's return a loan of £1 was made to him for immediate wants, which has been punctually repaid. Case was regularly visited, and it is hoped that influence brought to bear will make the man more careful in the future.

In a few instances assistance by way of the loan of a machine is desirable. It is usual in these instances to mark the machine as the property of the Society until the loan is paid. Cases have occurred in which the question of the exemption of the machine has been raised, when a distress has been levied on the borrower. When a distress is levied, the wearing apparel of the person or defendant and ot his family, and the tools and implements of his trade to the value of £5, are exempted from seizure. (*Cf.* 9 & 10 Vict., c. 95, and Law of Distress Amendment Act 1888.) But when distress is levied owing to non-payment of rent, the tenant loses this privilege (1) ' where the lease, term, or interest of the tenant has expired; (2) possession of the premises has been demanded; and (3) the distress is made 'not earlier than seven days after such demand.' *See* Stone's Justices' Manual, p. 538.]

Loans of machines, etc.

LXII.—Pensions.

Charity has to use the most determined efforts to replace the distressed in independence. There is one class of cases, however, in which such efforts would be thrown away, but for which, notwithstanding, assistance must be found. They are chronic or pension cases, in which misfortune has reduced a poor person to want, in spite of provision for the future and continued thrift, or when some special cause, such as the care of an aged or afflicted relation, has diminished the means of saving; or, again, when confirmed ill-health has made it impossible that the patient should earn a living, and yet it is not a case that should be left to the infirmary.

When pensions should be given.

A power recently granted to the Guardians of subscribing, with the consent of the Local Government Board, 'towards any asylum or institution for persons suffering from any permanent or natural infirmity or towards any association or society for aiding such persons ' [1] is important.

There is a great temptation to give pensions to respectable old people, without reference to any special conditions or qualifications. When there is a plain, private and personal responsibility on the part of the donor to relieve such persons by a pension, no objection can be raised to this being done; but when there is no such responsibility, and the onus of decision and relief rests upon those who have associated themselves together for charitable purposes,

[1] 42 & 43 Vict., c. 54, s. 10 *(see* p. cvi.).

some limitations are necessary, otherwise the pensions will tend to weaken providence and family ties, and to become an ill-regulated system of allowances, not unlike outdoor relief. The difficulty of procuring the necessary assistance and of providing sufficient personal supervision, must in any case, however, put a check on the granting of pensions, but the need of scrutiny thus enforced is beneficial.

The following general conditions may be suggested :—

1. That the pensioner should be of good general character.

2. That he should be over 60 years of age, except in cases in which he has been incapacitated by some serious accident or severe affliction. In every instance a medical certificate should be obtained.

3. That he should be unable to support himself by his own exertions.

4. That he should have made reasonable efforts to provide for old age. Due allowance would, of course, be made for exceptional difficulties against which he may have had to contend.

5. That relatives, employers, or others on whom he has either a legal or a strong moral claim, should join in assisting him.

6. That the pension should be sufficient to enable the recipient to live decently and in moderate comfort. For a couple, one shilling a day may perhaps be taken as a maximum adequate allowance for maintenance ; for single men or women, 8d. a day. In each case the rent must be allowed for in addition.

7. That the allowance be taken to the home weekly by an almoner.

8. That it should be revised every quarter, and any alterations in the condition of the pensioner, his means, and resources, may be ascertained and considered.

If granted in the first instance out of a kind of favouritism, and disbursed without constant personal supervision, pensions may entice the poor to manifold small deceits and pretences. Pensioners may, for instance, receive aid from others, even outdoor relief, and hide the fact that they are doing so. It is as with loans and much other relief; friendly watchfulness on the part of the almoner is indispensable.

For some cases in which the pensioners are, owing to old age and infirmity, unable to look after themselves, it is very difficult to make provision. An effort has to be made to procure for them admission to some one of the comparatively few suitable homes mentioned in the Register, or to board them out, if possible, with friends and relations. Very often in these cases the old people are best cared for in an infirmary.

The following cases may be quoted as illustrative :—

J. and M. G. are 66 and 64 years old. The man was a club (kitchen) porter, and his wife did nursing. Their earnings were never great, and they suffered the loss of all their six children. But they kept straight and saved £111. When the man became past work, this was spent. The woman still earns 2s. a week for charing, which has been supplemented by an allowance of 9s.

M. S., aged 72, was left a widow a year ago. She was married very young. The husband's earnings were always small. They had six children, of whom they had to bury two. In later years the man became very infirm, and could only earn a few shillings. He was insured, and the widow received £15. She still does a little washing, and friends and relations allow 3s. 6d. in small sums. The Committee have raised 2s. 6d. a week in addition.

T., a French governess, aged 63, had been unfit for any employment for 11 years, through illness, and had been supported by an elder brother who was an artist, who, through old age and reduced circumstances, could not continue to support her, further than giving her a home; she bore an excellent character, and had assisted to support her mother till her death. She had been engaged in good families, and we communicated with them, with the result that a pension of £40 a year for three years has been promised.

And, as an instance of a case of chronic illness, provided for by a pension, the following may be cited :—

U. V.—The case of a young woman suffering from what is certified to be incurable disease is taken up zealously by the clergy of the district in which she resides; the Committee is asked to endorse with its approval a special appeal which was to be printed and widely circulated. With the approval of the Central Office, after due inquiry, and under carefully considered conditions of administration, this endorsement was made; money has come to hand, which allows an adequate treatment of the case for a period beyond the probable duration of the young woman's life, and the amount is lodged with us under an agreement prepared in concert with the clergy.

LXIII.—Means of Thrift.

Charity's better work, however, is to induce the people to provide themselves with pensions. This can most readily be done by the friendly and benefit societies, and savings and post-office banks, post-office annuities, etc. Particulars regarding these will be found in the Appendix to the Register.[1] The almoner can always give relief on his own conditions, and one of the conditions should be that the father of the family and the children, as they grow up, should join a good friendly society.

How thrift can be made a condition of help.

It must often be the hope of the almoner that the rising generation will enjoy a better and completer life than their parents, one less harassed by the struggle for necessaries, and thus less exposed to mischance. If they begin by receiving the better instruction of the School Board schools, and are accustomed to think of thrift as one of the duties of life, there is a reasonable prospect of their making a step upwards. The boys, when they have left school, may join juvenile friendly societies. The number of these is rapidly increasing. The Manchester Unity of Odd Fellows have now in connection with their society 1,421 juvenile societies, with a membership of 90,057, and funds amounting to £95,569. In connection with the Foresters are 1,592 juvenile societies, with a membership (male and female) of 112,227, and funds amounting to £144,888. The Hearts of Oak have a juvenile society of 9,087 members, with a reserve fund of £11,924. In these societies, for a small payment, provision is made against sickness and funeral expenses, and there is no reason why, in a short time, old age should not be as satisfactorily provided for on a sound basis on insurances begun at the ages when lads usually become members. Clubs like these might draw their members from the schools, members who have acquired the habit of saving when young, and

Juvenile Friendly Societies.

[1] Particulars respecting existing arrangements will be found in the Post Office Guide.

are likely to stick to the society they join. Girls might leave school with a Post Office or Penny Bank banking account. At present, at least, there are not many friendly societies available for them. The School Board can, however, open savings banks in connection with the Post Office, and many of the schools have savings banks.

LXIV.—Friendly Societies.

Many of those who fall into distress do not belong to clubs.

Counts have frequently been made of the proportion of men who belong to clubs among those who apply for charitable relief. More recent data could be furnished, but the extract that we quote from the report of the St. Olave's Committee of the Charity Organisation Society for 1880 is still of interest, and indicates the great need of a large class of applicants in this respect. It must be remembered, however, that since then there has been a considerable increase in the membership of friendly societies. The Committee state that, out of 447 cases on their books in one year, 140 were casual labourers. 'Of these 99 were not members of any club or benefit society—that is, were making no provision whatever in case of sickness or death. Of the remaining, 15 belonged to clubs, 10 to slate clubs, and 16 had lost their clubs through not keeping up their payments. Such statistics,' the Report proceeds—

'must not of course be taken as affording any accurate testimony. But it is sufficiently clear that little can be done for a class where the most common form of providence does not prevail, and where the circumstances of their labour seem to foster vices which carry such hard consequences. As a further illustration we may note the fact that only 25 of the 447 were men engaged in the leather trade, which is carried on so extensively in Bermondsey. Of these 11 were members of a club, 8 were without a club, and 6 had been struck off for non-payment. It may be worth while to add that among the 447 consecutive cases examined there were 10 shoemakers (8 without a club), 8 painters (6 without a club), 7 clerks (6 without a club), 3 tailors (all without a club), 10 hawkers (all without a club). The importance of the sick club is generally acknowledged. Numerous applications for aid are made owing to sickness, where membership in a club would have insured a weekly payment of 18s. (Hearts of Oak), 14s. (Foresters), and so on. The Committee have therefore made their grant of relief conditional on the applicant undertaking to join a club, when age rendered it possible. H. F., a labourer, aged 28, married, two children, applied in February last for assistance. He had been an out-patient at Guy's Hospital for five weeks, had then poisoned his hand, by which he was kept from work for nine weeks more. He belonged to no club, and had therefore nothing to fall back on except credit and the pawnshop. Having stated that he had now a promise of regular work, which was confirmed by the foreman, the Committee made him a loan of 1l. 10s. to take some things out of pawn, also a grant of 15s. for relief, as his work did not begin at once, the latter sum being also advanced on loan, but with the further agreement that repayment would not be demanded if he joined a club. He paid back the loan at the rate of 2s. 6d. a week, commencing one month after he had been in work, and on September 27 joined the Comical Fellows' Benefit Society, paying an entrance fee of 5s.'

Tests of the soundness of clubs.

So much does the fact of being the member of a club say for a man, that it may be considered always a strong point in his favour in any application for assistance. And great good may be done by enabling men to pay their arrears. The members of some lodges, in times of pressure especially, will, on cause shown, pay up arrears in good cases. If a man states that he is 'run out,' the club card, if it be forthcoming, will show what the facts are; and the secretaries of the branches are generally willing to give information on such a point.

Sometimes, however, there is an apprehension that the club to which a man belongs is not financially sound. And hearing from time to time of failures of small clubs or lodges, an almoner hesitates to recommend a man to join a club, for fear lest it should swallow up his savings and even destroy his faith in the desirability of saving altogether. The mere registration of a society must not be considered as a guarantee of its trustworthiness. The number of members, the total assets and the yearly income of the club may be compared, so as to ascertain, by a kind of rule of thumb, the stability of the club. Short of an actuarial investigation, there is no other method so far as we know. In conjunction with the points that we have mentioned, a knowledge of the *bona fides* of the managers of the club is probably as good an assurance of stability as any. It may be considered safe to urge a man to join one of the three or four leading friendly societies, such as the Odd Fellows, the Foresters, or the Hearts of Oak. If he is too old, or cannot 'pass the doctor,' he may be able to provide for himself under one of the post office tables.[1]

The continuous growth of the large federated societies, which have at each decade reached a higher standard of administration as their members have realised more clearly the nature of the problems of insurance which each society was striving to solve, is one of the best guarantees of the future independence of the great mass of the working classes, for in these societies are to be found alike agricultural labourers and town artisans. In 'The Law of Friendly Societies,' edited by the Chief Registrar, Mr. Brabrook, will be found a short sketch of the progress of legislation in regard to these societies.[2] We quote the last paragraph, as it contains a warning which cannot be too often insisted on :—

'A word of caution may be added against forming too hasty conclusions adverse to friendly societies, from the fact that the valuations in many cases show an estimated deficiency in the funds to meet the liabilities. It would be strange if it were otherwise, when scientific tests are applied to contracts that have been in operation without a scientific basis for a long series of years. It must be borne in mind, however, that nothing is more elastic than the contract made by a friendly society with its members; no error more easy of remedy, if found out in time, than one existing

---

[1] *See* Post Office Guide.
[2] 'The Law of Friendly Societies,' Twelfth Edition. Shaw & Sons, Fetter Lane. 1894.

in the original terms of such a contract. Hence the words "insolvency," "rottenness," and the like, which we sometimes hear freely used as describing the general condition of friendly societies, are utterly out of place. Of friendly societies in general it may be said there are no associations the benefits of which are more important to their members; so there are none that are managed with greater rectitude, and few with equal success.'

LXV.—The Friendly Societies' Registry.

For what purposes friendly societies established. By the Friendly Societies Acts [1] there may be registered at the central office of the Friendly Societies Registry, 28 Abingdon Street, S.W.:

(1) Societies (herein called friendly societies) established to provide by voluntary subscriptions of members thereof, with or without aid of donations :—

'For the relief or maintenance of members, their husbands, wives, children, fathers, mothers, brothers or sisters, nephews or nieces, or wards being orphans, during sickness or other infirmity, whether bodily or mental, in old age (which shall mean any age after fifty), or in widowhood, or for the relief or maintenance of the orphan children of members during minority;

'For insuring money to be paid on the birth of a member's child, or on the death of a member, or for the funeral expenses of the husband, wife, or child of a member, or of the widow of a deceased member, or as respects persons of the Jewish persuasion, for the payment of a sum of money during the period of confined mourning;

'For the relief or maintenance of the members when on travel in search of employment, or when in distressed circumstances, or in case of shipwreck, or loss or damage of or to boats or nets;

'For the endowment of members or nominees of members at any age;

'For the insurance against fire to any amount not exceeding fifteen pounds of the tools or implements of the trade or calling of the members;

'Provided that no society (except as aforesaid) which contracts with any person for the assurance of an annuity exceeding fifty pounds per annum, or of a gross sum exceeding two hundred pounds, shall be registered under this Act.'

(2) Cattle insurance societies.

(3) Societies for any benevolent or charitable purpose.

(4) Societies (herein called working men's clubs) for the purposes of social intercourse, mutual happiness, mental and moral improvement, and rational recreation.

(5) Specially authorised societies.

The central office for registration, etc. The central office has to prepare and circulate forms of accounts, etc., for the use of societies, to collect returns, to publish information regarding statistics of life and sickness, and their application to the business of friendly societies; to publish from time to time generally, or in particular districts, such particulars of their returns and valuations, and such other information useful to members of, and persons interested in, friendly societies; to construct and publish tables for the payment of sums of money on

38 & 39 Vict., c. 60; 50 & 51 Vict., c. 56; 51 & 52 Vict., c. 66.

death, in sickness, or old age, etc. The Chief Registrar has to report yearly to Parliament.

The conditions required of societies that register and the forms to be filled up can be had on application to the Registrar.

A registration of a society fraudulently registered may be cancelled or suspended. Registered societies must have a registered office, must appoint trustees, whose appointment has to be notified to the Registrar, and must have its accounts audited annually by 'one of the public auditors appointed under the Act, or by two or more persons appointed as the rules of the society provide.' Societies registered before 1876 can be converted into the branches of other registered societies.[1] An annual return has to be made to the Registrar of the 'receipts and expenditure, funds, and effects, of the society as audited,' and 'the expenditure in respect of the several objects of the society'; the name and address and calling of the auditor have also to be given if the public auditor does not audit. Any member or person having an interest in the funds of the society may inspect the books, and, on application, have gratuitously a copy of the last annual return. The last balance-sheet, auditor's report, and quinquennial return has to be 'always hung up in a conspicuous place at the registered office.' A quinquennial valuation of assets and liabilities has to be made.

The privileges of the societies are, amongst others, that they may hold land in the names of their trustees; that they are exempt from stamp duty; that they have priority of claim in respect of money or property belonging to them in the possession of an officer by virtue of his office; and that a member of a friendly society who is 16 years of age can nominate a husband, wife, father, mother, child, brother, sister, nephew, or niece, or any other person who is not an officer or servant of the society, to receive on his death moneys due to him not exceeding £100 by authorisation sent to the registered office; and that in the event of a member of a society entitled to a sum not exceeding £100 dying without having made a nomination and intestate, the sum shall be payable without letters of administration to the person who appears to the majority of the trustees upon such evidence as they may deem satisfactory to be entitled by law to receive it. Persons above the age of 16 and less than 21 may enjoy all the rights of a member, execute instruments and give acquittances, but they cannot be members of the committee of management, trustees, managers, or treasurers. Societies consisting wholly of members of any age under 21, or exceeding these years, are allowed to register under special regulations. Members may obtain certificates of birth, death, etc., at 1s., paying 6d. for subsequent copies. The society may subscribe to 'any hospital, infirmary, charitable or provident institution, which may be necessary to secure to

[1] 39 & 40 Vict., c. 32, s. 3.

members and their families the benefit ' of such institutions—a proviso that might prove useful were medical benefits extended to the families of members.

Societies have to invest in post-office savings banks, or in any savings bank certified under the Act of 1863; in the public funds, with the Commissioners for the Reduction of the National Debt; in the purchase of land and erection of buildings; and in any other security expressly directed by the rules of the society, not being personal security, except as hereinafter authorised with respect to loans.

With regard to loans to members, not more than one-half of the amount of an assurance on the life of a member of at least one full year's standing may be advanced to him, on the written security of himself and two satisfactory securities for repayment. The societies may have separate loan funds formed of the contributions and deposits of members. They may then make loans to members on their personal security, with or without sureties, according to the society's rules. But (amongst other restrictions) the loan cannot be made out of money contributed for other purposes. No member can hold any interest in a loan fund exceeding £200. No loan without security may, together with moneys owing by the member, exceed £50. Officers have to give security if required by the rules. For the purpose of legal proceedings, a society is represented by the trustees, and in some instances the officers.

Members, or persons claiming through members, are not entitled to receive more than £200 by way of gross sum, together with any bonuses or additions declared upon assurances not exceeding that amount, or (excepting in the case of societies established before 1850, in which a larger sum could be claimed) more than £50 a year from any one or more such societies. Societies may not insure, or pay on the death of a child under five years of age, any sum of money, which added to the amount payable on the death of such child by any other society exceeds £6. Nor may they insure or pay on the death of a child under 10 years of age any sum which, with similar additions, exceeds £10. The sum has to be paid to the parent or his representative, on the production of a certificate of death in a prescribed form.

Poor Law relief, as has been shown, is intended for the destitute. Therefore it has to provide what is sufficient to prevent destitution, and no more. If the applicant has means, but means insufficient for his maintenance, the Guardians have to make it up to the standard of ' necessary relief.' Properly speaking, any moneys received from relations, savings, benefits drawn from a friendly society should be treated as income, though, possibly, income insufficient to prevent destitution. But the Legislature has been inclined to give privileges to members of friendly societies. One such privilege is that, in cases in which the member of a friendly society comes on the rates, his club allowance may be reserved for the maintenance of his wife or other relative dependent on him, instead of being paid towards his own maintenance. The other privilege is that the Guardians may, if they think fit, do more than prevent destitution in the case of members of friendly societies to whom they decide to give relief. They may relieve them without taking their club money into account.

'Notwithstanding any orders or regulations of the Poor Law Commissioners or the Local Government Board under and by virtue of the Poor Law Amendment Act 1834,[1] or of any Act amending the said Act, it shall be lawful for any Board of Guardians, if they think fit, to grant relief out of the poor rates to any person otherwise entitled to such relief, notwithstanding that the said person shall, by reason of his membership of a friendly society, be in receipt of any sum, and that, in estimating the amount of the relief that shall be granted to such person being a member of a friendly society as aforesaid, it shall be at the discretion of the Board of Guardians whether they will or will not take into consideration the amount which may be received by him from such friendly society.'[2]

This Act does not extend to Scotland or Ireland.

If a pauper or pauper lunatic, having a wife or other relative dependent upon him for maintenance, be entitled to receive moneys as a member of any friendly or benefit society, such moneys shall, subject to any deductions required for keeping up his membership, be paid or applied by the trustees, committee, or officers of the society, to or for the maintenance of such wife or relative. If a pauper or pauper lunatic, having no wife or relative dependent on him, is so entitled, no claim shall be made on the society by the Guardians, 'unless and until' they or their 'relieving officer shall have declared the relief to be given on loan, and shall have, within thirty days thereof, notified the same in writing to the secretary or trustees of the society or branch of which the pauper or pauper lunatic is a member.'[3]

'Where the rules allowed certain benefits in cases of sickness, it was held that "insanity" was within the meaning of the term "sickness." But where the rules provided that a member falling sick, lame, or blind, or otherwise disabled for work, should be entitled to a certain weekly allowance, it was held that incapacity for work, arising from natural decay by the result of old age, did not entitle a member to the allowance.'[4]

LXVI.—Post Office Arrangements for Thrift and Saving.[5]

The Post Office authorities have recently published a short paper on the advantages furnished to depositors by the Post Office Savings Banks, which are under Government security. The almoner

[1] 4 & 5 Will. IV., c. 76.
[2] Out-door Relief Friendly Societies Act 1894, 57 & 58 Vict., c. 25.
[3] 42 Vict., c. 12, amending 39 & 40 Vict., c. 61, s. 23 (1879).
[4] 'Poor Law Statutes,' Macmorran. Vol. IV., p. 12 (1890).
[5] A list of savings banks will be found in the Register.

will find further information in the Postal Guide, which is published quarterly, price 6d., and can be had at any Post Office :—

'Post Office Savings Banks—Advantages to Depositors.

'*Security.*—The Post Office Savings Banks are established by Act of Parliament, and every depositor has the *direct security* of the State for the repayment of his deposits.

'*Hours of Business.*—Post Office Savings Banks are open for the receipt of deposits on week days during the hours appointed for the sale of stamps. Every such office is also open for the payment of withdrawals on week days during certain hours which are specified in a notice exhibited at the office.

'*Deposits.*—Any sum from a shilling upwards, excluding pence, may be deposited at one time, and any number of deposits may be made in the course of a year (ending December 31) up to a limit of £50. A person may have £200 in all on his deposit account, including interest.

'*Withdrawals* can be made with the utmost promptitude by sending notice by post to the London chief office on the form provided for the purpose, which is obtainable at any Post Office Savings Bank, and payment can be received at any Post Office Savings Bank in the United Kingdom convenient to the depositor without regard to the office of deposit.

'During any year ending December 31, a depositor may replace the amount of any one withdrawal previously made in the same year.

'*Withdrawals by Telegraph.*—On application at any Post Office Savings Bank which is also a telegraph office, and on producing the deposit book, a depositor may, by paying the cost of the necessary telegrams, obtain payment on the day of notice of any sum up to £10, or payment can be received by return of post of any sum up to £20. Application should be made between 9 a.m. and 4 p.m. (Saturdays, 9 a.m. and 1 p.m.)

'*Interest* at the rate of £2. 10s. per cent. per annum is allowed on every complete pound deposited so long as the sum to a depositor's credit does not exceed £200. Whenever the balance exceeds that sum, interest will be allowed on £200, and the excess will be invested for the depositor in Government stock unless the depositor should otherwise direct.

'*Small Savings by Stamps.*—Forms, with spaces for 12 penny stamps, intended for the use of persons desirous of saving one shilling by means of penny contributions for deposit in the Post Office Savings Bank, can be obtained at any post office in the United Kingdom.

'*Children's Deposits.*—Money may be deposited by children who have attained the age of seven years, and also on behalf and in the names of children under that age. Depositors over seven years of age are entitled to deal with their deposits in the same manner as persons of full age, but children under seven years of age cannot withdraw their deposits until they have reached the age of seven.

'*Societies and Penny Banks.*—Deposits may be made by friendly societies, by charitable or provident institutions or societies, and by penny savings banks, provided application be first made to the Controller of the Savings Bank Department, accompanied by a copy of the rules. Deposits may also be made by corporate bodies and corporations sole. Certain societies, &c., are allowed to invest considerably beyond the usual limit, and some without restriction as to amount, according to circumstances. Especial aid is given to penny banks established in connection with the Post Office Savings Bank.

'*Transfer from a Trustee Savings Bank.*—If a depositor in a trustee savings bank wishes to place his money in a Post Office Savings Bank, he should apply to the trustees of the savings bank for a certificate of transfer (in the form prescribed by the 10th section of the Act 24 Vict., c. 14), and should pay the certificate into any Post Office Savings Bank as if it were a cheque. By adopting this course, the depositor will avoid trouble and the risk of carrying cash from one bank to the other.

'*Depositor's Book can be used at any Post Office Savings Bank.*—A depositor may add to his deposits, or withdraw the whole or any part of them, at any Post Office Savings Bank in the United Kingdom, without change of deposit book.

' *Nominations.* A depositor of the age of 16 years, or upwards, may, subject to certain limits, nominate any person to receive his savings bank deposits at death. A form for the purpose may be obtained, free of cost, from the Controller of the Savings Bank Department.

' *Secrecy.*—The strictest secrecy is observed with respect to the names and addresses of depositors in Post Office Savings Banks, and the amounts deposited or withdrawn by them.

' *Postage Free.*—No charge for postage is made to a depositor, if in the United Kingdom, for any letter passing between him and the chief office on Post Office Savings Bank business.

' FACILITIES FOR INVESTING IN THE FUNDS.

' *Investments in Government Stock* can be made through any Post Office Savings Bank of sums from one shilling to £200 stock in any year ending December 31, until the maximum of £500 stock has been reached; and money can be deposited for this purpose irrespective of ordinary savings bank deposits. The dividends are collected by the Post Office and added to the depositors' accounts without charge.

' *Sales.*—A depositor who buys stock in this way can sell the whole or a part of it at any time through the Post Office Savings Bank.

' *Commission.*—The commission on a purchase or a sale of stock is 9*d.* for stock not exceeding £25, and 6*d.* on each further £25 up to £100. Beyond this it is 6*d.* more for each additional £100 stock or part of £100 stock.

' *Further Provisions in regard to Stock.*—A depositor may, at a small cost, transfer stock into his name at the Bank of England, or obtain a stock certificate with dividend coupons annexed.'

One paragraph from the Postal Guide, in regard to the persons by whom deposits may be made, we quote :—

' Deposits may be made—

'(A) By persons of full age, and not under legal disability.

'(B) By married women.

'(C) By children seven years old and upwards.

'(D) On behalf and in the names of children under 7 years old. In this case the money is not repayable until the children attain the age of 7, except in the event of death.

'(E) On behalf of insane persons by those appointed to represent them.

'(F) By two or more persons jointly on their own behalf, provided no one of them has any other account in a savings bank, and the signature of both persons will be required to a notice of withdrawal.

'(G) By one person as trustee for another person also named in the account. A person may act as trustee in any number of accounts, and at the same time have an account in his own name.

' (H) By a duly registered friendly society through its trustees. In this case deposits may be made without limit.

'(I) By a duly registered industrial and provident society not chargeable with income tax. In this case deposits may be made without limit.

'(J) By a charitable or provident society, penny bank, or similar institution, through the trustees or treasurer. In this case deposits may be made to the extent of £100 in any one year, and £300 in the whole, and, if the consent of the National Debt Commissioners be obtained, without limit.

'(K) By societies, limited companies, and other corporations not coming under (H), (I), or (J). In these cases the ordinary limits for deposits, as explained above under "Deposits" (*see* clause 3, "Post Office Savings Bank," in Postal Guide), apply.

'(L) By vicars and rectors of parishes and other official persons, being corporations sole, in their official titles. In these cases the ordinary limits apply.

'(M) In the name of the registrar of any County Court. Under the 70th section of the County Courts Act, 51 & 52 Vict., c. 43. "trust moneys" not in excess of £500 may be thus deposited; and under the 71st section, money paid into a County Court in "equitable proceedings" may be deposited by the registrar without restriction as to amount.

'When it is desired to deposit under (H), (I), or (J), application must first be made for authority to the Controller of the Savings Bank Department, accompanied by a copy of rules.

'Special facilities are provided for assisting managers of penny banks and for the saving of pence by children attending elementary schools. Full information will be furnished on application to the Controller of the Savings Bank Department.'

In connection with the public elementary schools in London, there are many school savings banks.

LXVII.—THE COLLECTING SAVINGS BANK.

The Collecting Savings Bank.

As a means of reaching the labouring class and drawing them into habits of thrift and saving, the Collecting Savings Bank will be found useful, but its usefulness will depend on its being dissociated from relief work and on regularity in collection. It should assume the character of a business, and it cannot be too strongly insisted that the Collecting Savings Bank should be chiefly a stepping-stone to some other kind of thrift—a savings bank account, membership of a friendly society, etc. The following extracts are taken from a paper published by the London Charity Organisation Society :—

'Probably in every parish or district in England there exists some organisation for collecting money for special purposes, such as coal, clothing clubs, &c., but the distinctive feature of collecting banks is that they are for saving pure and simple, the money when saved being absolutely at the disposal of the depositor.

'Without doubt the Post Office Savings Bank, offering as it does a fair rate of interest combined with absolute security, is well adapted to meet the requirements of the naturally thrifty and better educated class of skilled artisans; but as regards the uneducated and poorer class of workpeople, it has remained almost a dead letter. There are other savings banks where depositors may place a humbler amount than the 1s. required by the Post Office, but experience shows that there are great numbers of the people who, either through ignorance or shiftlessness, will not make use of any of the ordinary channels for saving. They will go to no savings bank. In the first instance, at any rate, *the savings bank must go to them.*

'It is here that the collecting bank steps in, the small amount that can well be spared, but would never have found its way to any savings bank, being intercepted, as it were, before the wage-earner has let it slip through his fingers.

'This is not an ideal state of things, and it is highly desirable, where a Collecting Savings Bank is established, that depositors should be led on to place their savings either with the Post Office or some other well-established bank, instead of making their thrift dependent upon the weekly visit of the collector. For this reason it is better not to allow any interest or bonus whatever upon the money collected.[1]

'The usual method of starting a collecting bank is for some responsible persons known in the district to introduce to the people those who propose to undertake

---

[1] The largest collecting societies, viz., those of Liverpool and Manchester, and others who follow on their lines, allow no interest. It does not appear that those which give interest flourish better than those which do not.

the collection, and inform them upon what day and at about what time the collector will call; or sometimes notices are distributed giving the same information and stating the objects of the bank. The collector gives to each depositor a card ruled on one side, so as to allow the entering of a payment for every week in the year, and on the other the rules of the bank are printed. Upon a payment being made, it is the business of the collector to enter it upon the card and also in a book kept for that purpose. It is very advisable that there should be more than one person responsible for the money collected and general management of the bank, not only as a precaution against the possible contingency of fraud (although this is not to be overlooked), but chiefly because, should there be but one person responsible, and he were to die or meet with an accident rendering him incapable of attending to the affairs of the bank, the depositors might be placed in a very awkward position. It must be borne in mind that any hitch, such as delay in repaying deposits, &c., is destructive of confidence, and may be a serious matter to the humble depositor.

'The best time for visiting the houses for collecting purposes is in the early part of the week (Monday morning being quite the best time); but whatever day may be arranged, it is highly important that the collection should be made *regularly*, as experience shows that if a week be missed the money that would have been saved is hardly ever forthcoming the following week.

'The money collected should at once be handed over to the person responsible for the management of the bank, and it is very desirable that all sums collected should be paid into the Post Office Savings Bank to an account opened for that purpose, both as a precaution of safety and also because the interest obtained, even if of a very small amount, will go far towards defraying the trifling expenses of printing, &c.

'It will be found that in most cases the bulk of the money deposited is drawn out before Christmas, the depositors starting again early in the new year. But although this is not satisfactory, yet the fact that the depositor has something in hand during the year to meet his requirements and need not run into debt is a point gained for the cause of thrift, and may lead to a better state of things. An important feature of this collecting system is the opportunity which it gives of bringing to the knowledge of working people the advantages offered by the Post Office Savings Bank and by the various friendly and other societies which exist for their benefit.

'The work of collecting is but slight. Two hours a week will do a great deal, and with fair organisation a large district can be worked by a few collectors.

'Another plan which has been found by well-known and experienced workers to be useful is that of the sale of stamps, to be affixed to the forms supplied by the Post Office. When a form is filled up by the twelve stamps required, the visitor is able to open a Post Office Savings Bank account, which can be constantly added to in the name of the depositor. The advantages of this plan are (1) that the visitor becomes a link between the depositor and the Post Office Savings Bank, and (2) that no book-keeping is necessary.

'Collectors should be strictly forbidden to give anything in the shape of relief, either in money or goods.

'All collectors who have had experience can relate instances where the humble start made in the Collecting Savings Bank has led to permanent habits of thrift and to prosperity.'

LXVIII.—EXCEPTIONAL DISTRESS.

The following suggestions were formulated by a Special Committee in 1886, and may be found useful in times of emergency.

SUGGESTIONS AND SUGGESTED RULES FOR DEALING WITH EXCEPTIONAL DISTRESS BY LOCAL COMMITTEES.

I. GENERAL POLICY OF RELIEF.

It has now been repeatedly proved that the only way to meet wide-spread and exceptional distress, without doing permanent injury to the mass of the poor, is to adhere to certain general principles and fixed lines of action which they will readily understand. Indecision and vacillation at such a time produce grave mischief.[1]

The creation of a large relief fund tends to occasion additional difficulties and perplexities. Confusion and waste can only be avoided by taking careful measures for the administration of relief beforehand, quietly and without panic.

'Tests' and inquiry.

To deal with large numbers of people quickly and effectually 'tests' are necessary, no less than inquiry.

Classes requiring relief.

Roughly speaking, applications come from three classes :

(1) Thrifty and careful men ;

(2) Men of different grades of respectability, with a decent home ;

(3) The idle, loafing class, or those brought low by drink or vice.

To the first of these, relief should be given ; but if public works are opened they should be recommended to take such work, not as a test, but as temporary employment.

To the second class (according to the character of the case) relief should be offered (1) conditionally on employment in public or other works ; or (2) the applicant should be referred to the Poor Law labour-yard ; or (3) admitted to the workhouse, while the wife and family are supported by charitable relief outside.

The third class should be left to the Poor Law. Relief by way of alms only maintains them in their evil habits, discourages the thrifty and striving, and leads to still further neglect of wife and family.

Public and charitable 'works.'

Public works should not be undertaken unless there is clear evidence that the want of employment is so great that some such temporary measures are absolutely necessary to prevent better-class working men from living in semi-starvation. Their tendency must be to keep labour in the same grooves. If the distress is occasioned by some temporary and definite cause, after a short period there

---

[1] 'On the best means of dealing with Exceptional Distress ; the report of a Special Committee of the Charity Organisation Society, 1886.' Much evidence on the subject, and particulars regarding the agencies and methods of relief, etc., will be found in the Report.

In a time of 'commercial embarrassment' 'an ill-regulated distribution of charitable donations may not only fail to relieve the class for whose benefit the funds were collected, but further diminish the resources they would otherwise have obtained by their own exertions.'— Dr. Kay, Third Annual Report of the Poor Law Commissioners.

'It is the stoutest, not the kindest, heart that is wanted' 'in times of scarcity or unusual stagnation' ; and 'all we have to do is to weather the storm as well as we are able, taking additional care to be vigilant and strict in keeping all members of the community within the bounds of duty.'—Quoted by Mr. Longley in his 'Report to the Local Government Board on Poor Law Administration in London,' 1874.

will be an improvement in the labour market. If the distress is occasioned by deeper and more permanent causes, public works will act merely as a palliative which may divert attention from the source of the evil and tend to become as chronic as the shortness of work.

If public or other works are opened—

(1) Men should only be admitted to them after inquiry or on satisfactory recommendation.

(2) The wages and the hours should be as nearly as possible according to contract rates; and the work should be piece-work, given out and paid for according to measure.

(3) Care should be taken to supply sufficient overlookers, and to group the men according to character and ability.

(4) If a meal is wanted, or clothing, it is better that this should be supplied separately from a relief fund. The employment should be given, as far as possible, in accordance with ordinary business contracts, and not as ' charity work,' which tends to be as ill-done as it is ill-paid, and to degrade men instead of improving them.

(5) Public and other relief works should be of a local character, planned according to estimates drawn by the local authorities, and conducted under local superintendence. This will be some guarantee against waste and irresponsibility. Such works only should be undertaken as are likely to create the least disturbance in the labour market.

Poor Law Labour-yards are sometimes the only test available, but they have a tendency to become permanent institutions for the supply of cheaply paid and practically useless labour to casual and idle labourers of all kinds. Labour-yards.

The plan of applying a modified form of the workhouse test in certain cases, by which the man is maintained in the workhouse while the wife and family are supported by voluntary charity, is suggested for the following reasons : The modified workhouse test.

(1) The assistance is adequate ; no homes are broken up, and the relief is so given as to meet the wants of the family—the wife and children as well as the husband.

(2) It will act as an education in provident habits.

(3) The burden of sacrifice will be thrown on the man : whereas in all other schemes for dealing with this class, it is liable to be thrown on the woman.

II. THE LOCAL COMMITTEES.

It is clear that none of the three classes mentioned above, except the first and part of the second, can be properly dealt with, unless there is co-operation between the administrators of charitable funds and the Poor Law Guardians. This co-operation is indispensable. Co-operation with Guardians indispensable.

Of whom they should consist.

That there may be agencies for this co-operation and for the direct distribution of relief, local Relief Committees are necessary. These should include representatives—

(*a*) Of the Principal Land and House Owners,

(*b*) Of Employers of Labour,

(*c*) Of Working Men—including representatives of trade societies and benefit clubs,

(*d*) Of charitable agencies,

(*e*) Of Poor Law Guardians and of the Vestry,

(*f*) Of School Teachers and Visitors,

(*g*) Of Clergy of all denominations.

Committees should be comparatively small and composed of members well acquainted with the district. To such persons the street or neighbourhood in which a man lives may be a rough test of some value. So far as possible, people of judgment, who have had some experience, and have already interested themselves in the work of charity, should be chosen. Members, *e.g.*, ought to know what questions to ask and how to take down an application. The Clergy should act as advisers to the Committee, rather than as almoners or honorary officials. Their knowledge of the district, of the persons who apply, is often very valuable.

Area of Committee.

The area covered by the Committee should be comparatively small.

How to avoid a rush.

To avoid a rush of cases—

(1) Unnecessary publicity should, in the earlier stages, be avoided.

(2) The rules which the Committee propose to follow should subsequently be advertised in local papers, and given to all applicants. These rules should show in general terms, but clearly, whom the Committee wish to relieve and whom they intend to leave to the Poor Law. (*See* paragraph iv.)

(3) It should be clearly stated that relief will only be given after inquiry, or with a labour test.

(4) Trustworthy persons, who have been selected for the purpose by the Committee, and who are well acquainted with the district, should refer to the Committee cases which they believe they can thoroughly recommend. A number of suitable cases may thus be brought to light, and the multitude of personal applications in part avoided.

III. INQUIRY.

Application on recommendations.

Applications should in all cases be made by the head of the family only.

Application forms, or forms of reference, should be given to members of Committee, selected employers and foremen, the officers of trade and benefit societies, and to clergymen and district visitors of experience.

These forms should be given by them to applicants whom they recommend as suitable, according to the rules. (*See* above.)

The applicant should be required to attend at the office, and bring with him the application or reference form, duly filled up and signed; and, if the person who sends the case is not an employer or foreman, a recommendation from the employer or foreman will be necessary.

In all these cases the home will be visited and the reference or recommendation verified, if the pressure is too great to do more. If not, other points in the case may be taken up with a view to a more thorough treatment of it. *Direct application.*

If there is no reference of the applicant to the Committee, he will attend at the office, the application form will be filled up, and such inquiries made as the time allows.

Two things should never be omitted :—

(*a*) *The home should be visited.*

(*b*) *An employer or local reference should be communicated with.*

The inquiry should be made by members of Committees and others who have had some experience in relief work. They may in many instances require the assistance of one or more paid officers. It was found last year that much time was saved by the use of a form for corresponding with references or employers. *Who should make the inquiry.*

To ensure co-operation with the Guardians, it will be well to ascertain from them whether cases are known to them; and the Guardians might be asked to supply a list of the names of persons in receipt of parochial assistance. Similarly lists of those relieved by the Committee should be sent to the Guardians from time to time. *Inquiry of Relieving Officers.*

IV. DECISION.

To prevent delay and haphazard and unjust decisions, it will be found convenient to come to an understanding with regard to groups of cases; with this object it is suggested that the following rules should be adopted by the Committee, and only deviated from by vote on any special case. *Sifting of cases. Decisions.*

1. That persons known to be drunkards, 'loafers,' or persons of bad character, should not be assisted.[1]

2. That no one in receipt of Poor Law relief should be assisted, except by the payment of club arrears.

[1] This rule should be adhered to even when there is a wife and family. Otherwise the husband is encouraged to neglect them. Few persons realise how strong a feeling self-reliant working men have as to the waste and injustice of the relief thoughtlessly given to this class.

3. That no cases of chronic distress, in which the head of a family is habitually out of work in the winter or never in regular work, be assisted.

4. That no cases of chronic distress occasioned by long-continued illness, or by old age, be assisted.[1]

5. That no persons living in common lodging-houses should be assisted.

6. That relief should not be given to persons who have not resided in the district of the Poor Law Union for more than six months, unless there be special reason to the contrary.

7. That those who have made any provision for the future should be assisted.[2]

It should be remembered that for several of the above classes it will be best to apply some form of labour test, *e.g.* the labour-yard, etc. ; they would then obtain relief conditionally. But no applicants should be sent to public works, or works set on foot by any relief association, except on recommendation from some trustworthy source or after inquiry.

Decisions upon cases should be made by Committee, and not left to individual almoners.

Meetings. The Committee should meet daily, if possible. At least half the meetings should be held in the evening, so that working men may be able to attend.

V. RELIEF.

Suitable relief only possible if there is sufficient inquiry with trustworthy recommendation. Relief can be varied and adjusted to the actual wants of an applicant, only if the inquiry is sufficient or the person who recommends the case has a real knowledge of it. To minimise friction and delay and promote effective relief, these two means of discrimination---recommendation and inquiry---should be worked together.

Relief not given at office. *Relief should not be given at the office, but taken to the homes by members of Committee, almoners or others.* Valuable information is frequently obtained in this way, and crowding at the offices is still further prevented.

The visitor also may find that the relief ordered should be withheld for further instructions.

A receipt should be required in all cases upon the Application Form (see back of the Form).

Scale of relief. If, owing to the number of applications, it is not possible to adjust the relief to the wants of each case, the following scale, the sufficiency of which has been tested by experience, should be adopted as a minimum :

[1] These would naturally be dealt with by the more permanent relief agencies.
[2] Tests of this provision would be membership of a club or benefit society, membership of a trade society, savings as shown by bank book, &c.

Weekly Scale for Food and Fuel exclusive of Rent.

An adult living alone, 3s. 6d.

Two or more adults living together, 2s. 6d. each.

Children under 4 years, 6d. each.

 ,, from 4 to 12 years, 1s. each.

 ,, from 12 to 16 years, 1s. 6d. each.

Not more than 10s. in one week should, as a rule, be given to any family, as there are generally in large families earnings or income (other than charity) available.

Relief in kind is not recommended. It is no safeguard to give such relief in doubtful cases, cases in which the head of the family is a drunkard, or where the inquiry is defective. Knowledge of the case is the only real safeguard. Relief in kind.

If, however, relief is given in kind, it should be by orders on any respectable tradesman in the neighbourhood. An arbitrary and injurious interference with the custom of the smaller and poorer shopkeepers in the district will thus be avoided.

Soup-kitchens tend to bring masses of the poor together to be relieved wholesale. The chronic poor may be accustomed to this method of relief. Those of a better type, whom it is the problem of charity to relieve as far as possible, privately and without lowering their self-respect, will shrink from such distributions.

In special cases it may be found desirable to assist by providing meals. Orders upon cook and coffee shops, or coffee taverns, should then be given. It may be necessary to provide food for children in this way.

If clothing or boots are required, these too may be provided, after strict inquiry, and when there is definite promise of work.

If boots are given for children, inquiry should always be made of the schoolmaster or mistress in the first instance, and they should be informed of the gift.

As a rule it is best to take a view of the whole case, and to estimate its wants, with a view to its ultimate requirements; and then to give to the applicant in money what is necessary for his adequate assistance. If this be a temporary allowance, it will be given weekly.

If money is given for any special purpose, the visitor or almoner who has taken it should be required to report that it has been expended in the manner agreed upon with the applicant. He should see the receipts. Report of visitor as to use of money.

It is not desirable to pay the applicant's rent, if it can be avoided. But if, as is often the case, a portion of the relief will be used for the rent, it is better to recognise the fact and pay a week's current rent. Payment of rent.

Back rent should under no circumstances be paid.

The following further forms of relief are suggested :

(1) Payment of club arrears, after consultation with workmen upon the Committee, and reference to the Secretary of the Club, to whom the money should be paid.

(2) Taking tools and necessaries out of pawn. The money should in this case be paid to the pawnbroker direct.

(3) Medical relief.

(4) Migration.

(5) The emigration of carefully chosen emigrants to colonies in which it has been ascertained that there is a definite opening for them.

It has been found that many of the most distressing cases occur after a period of distress, and as the result of the privation and sickness which it causes. However large the fund, therefore, there should be no over-haste in distributing it. The money will be hardly less wanted some weeks after than at the actual time of the greatest pressure of applications. And it will be easier then to do justice to the work.

Cases after pressure is over.

APPENDIX.

EMPLOYERS' LIABILITY ACT.

It has been suggested that a note upon the Employers' Liability Act 1880) 51 & 52 Vict. c. 58) and continued since that date, would be of use. The following are its principal clauses :—

Amendment of law.
1. Where after the commencement of this Act personal injury is caused to a workman

(1.) By reason of any defect in the condition of the ways, works, machinery, or plant connected with or used in the business of the employer ; or

(2.) By reason of the negligence of any person in the service of the employer who has any superintendence entrusted to him whilst in the exercise of such superintendence ; or

(3.) By reason of the negligence of any person in the service of the employer to whose orders or directions the workman at the time of the injury was bound to conform, and did conform, where such injury resulted from his having so conformed ; or

(4) By reason of the act or omission of any person in the service of the employer done or made in obedience to the rules or byelaws of the employer, or in obedience to particular instructions given by any person delegated with the authority of the employer in that behalf; or

(5) By reason of the negligence of any person in the service of the employer who has the charge or control of any signal, points, locomotive engine, or train upon a railway,

the workman, or in case the injury results in death, the legal personal representatives of the workman, and any persons entitled in case of death, shall have the same right of compensation and remedies against the employer as if the workman had not been a workman of nor in the service of the employer, nor engaged in his work.

Exceptions to amendment of law.
2. A workman shall not be entitled under this Act to any right of compensation or remedy against the employer in any of the following cases ; that is to say,

(1) Under sub-section one of section one, unless the defect therein mentioned arose from, or had not been discovered or remedied owing to, the negligence of the employer, or of some person in the service of the

employer, and entrusted by him with the duty of seeing that the ways, works, machinery, or plant were in proper condition.

(2.) Under sub-section four of section one, unless the injury resulted from some impropriety or defect in the rules, byelaws, or instructions therein mentioned; provided that where a rule or a byelaw has been approved or has been accepted as a proper rule or byelaw by one of Her Majesty's Principal Secretaries of State, or by the Board of Trade or any other department of the Government, under or by virtue of any Act of Parliament, it shall not be deemed for the purposes of this Act to be an improper or defective rule or byelaw

(3.) In any case where the workman knew of the defect or negligence which caused his injury, and failed within a reasonable time to give, or cause to be given, information thereof to the employer or some person superior to himself in the service of the employer, unless he was aware that the employer or such superior already knew of the said defect or negligence.

3. The amount of compensation recoverable under this Act shall not exceed such sum as may be found to be equivalent to the estimated earnings during the three years preceding the injury, of a person in the same grade employed during those years in the like em.loyment and in the district in which the workman is employed at the time of the injury. *Limit of sum recoverable as compensation.*

4. An action for the recovery under this Act of compensation for an injury shall not be maintainable unless notice that injury has been sustained is given within six weeks, and the action is commenced within six months from the occurrence of the accident causing the injury, or, in case of death within twelve months from the time of death: Provided always, that in case of death the want of such notice shall be no bar to the maintenance of such action if the judge shall be of opinion that there was reasonable excuse for such want of notice. *Limit of time for recovery of compensation.*

5. There shall be deducted from any compensation awarded to any workman, or representatives of a workman, or persons claiming by, under, or through a workman in respect of any cause of action arising under this Act, any penalty or part of a penalty which may have been paid in pursuance of any other Act of Parliament to such workman, representatives, or persons in respect of the same cause of action; and where an action has been brought under this Act by any workman, or the representatives of any workman, or any persons claiming by, under, or through such workman, for compensation in respect of any cause of action arising under this Act, and payment has not previously been made of any penalty or part of a penalty under any other Act of Parliament in respect of the same cause of action, such workman, representatives, or person shall not be entitled thereafter to receive any penalty or part of a penalty under any other Act of Parliament in respect of the same cause of action. *Money payable under penalty to be deducted from compensation under Act.*

6.—(1.) Every action for recovery of compensation under this Act shall be brought in a county court, but may, upon the application of either plaintiff or defendant, be removed into a superior court in like manner and upon the same conditions as an action commenced in a county court may by law be removed. *Trial of actions.*

(2.) Upon the trial of any such action in a county court before the judge without a jury one or more assessors may be appointed for the purpose of ascertaining the amount of compensation.

(3.) For the purpose of regulating the conditions and mode of appointment and remuneration of such assessors, and all matters of procedure relating to their duties, and also for the purpose of consolidating any actions under this Act in a county court, and otherwise preventing multiplicity of such actions, rules and regulations may be made, varied, and repealed from time to time in the same manner as rules and regulations for regulating the practice and procedure in other actions in county courts.

8. For the purposes of this Act, unless the context otherwise requires,— *Definitions.*

The expression " person who has superintendence entrusted to him " means a person whose sole or principal duty is that of superintendence, and who is not ordinarily engaged in manual labour:

The expression " employer " includes a body of persons corporate or unincorporate:

The expression " workman " means a railway servant and any person to whom the Employers and Workmen Act, 1875, applies.　　*n 2*

BOOKS FOR REFERENCE & READING CONCERNING CHARITY
ND
QUESTIONS BEARING UPON CHARITABLE WORK.

The reader who desires to learn what grave issues depend on a right administration of the Poor Law and of charity cannot do better than study the Report of the Poor Law Commissioners, 1834. Chalmers' works; Edward Denison's Letters; Walker's Original will be found most useful and suggestive. We give a list, by no means exhaustive, of books which those who wish to learn something of the subject generally should read. There is a library at the offices of the Council of the Charity Organisation Society which contains a large number of books, pamphlets, returns, and reports which may be of use to students and inquirers.

I.—GENERAL.

THE REPORT OF THE POOR LAW COMMISSIONERS (1834). EXTRACTS from the information received by H.M. COMMISSIONERS as to the Administration and Operation of the Poor Laws (1837).

THE CHRISTIAN AND CIVIC ECONOMY OF LARGE TOWNS. By THOMAS CHALMERS, D.D. (1846).

Also ON THE SUFFICIENCY OF THE PAROCHIAL SYSTEM. By the same author.

THE ORIGINAL. By the late THOMAS WALKER, M.A. Fifth Edition. Edited, with Additions, by WM. A. GUY, M.B., F.R.S. Henry Renshaw, 356 Strand, London (1875).

LETTERS AND OTHER WRITINGS OF THE LATE EDWARD DENISON. Edited by Sir Baldwyn Leighton, Bart. London: Richard Bentley & Son (1875).

SOCIAL DUTIES, considered with reference to the organisation of effort in works of benevolence and public utility. London and Cambridge: Macmillan & Co. (1867).

*HOMES OF THE LONDON POOR. By OCTAVIA HILL. London: Macmillan & Co. (1884). Price 1s.

*OUR COMMON LAND. By OCTAVIA HILL. London: Macmillan & Co. (1877).

CONFESSIONS OF AN OLD ALMSGIVER. London: Wm. Hunt & Co. (1871).

THE THOUGHTS AND EXPERIENCES OF A CHARITY ORGANISA-TIONIST. By J. HORNSBY WRIGHT (1878).

METHOD IN ALMSGIVING. A Handbook for Helpers. By M. W. MOGGRIDGE. John Murray, Albemarle Street (1882). 3s. 6d.

THE MAKING OF THE HOME. A Reading Book of Domestic Economy. By Mrs. SAMUEL A. BARNETT. London: Cassell & Co.

THE DEAD HAND: Addresses on the subject of Endowments. By Lord HOBHOUSE, Q.C., K.C.S.I. London: Chatto & Windus, Piccadilly (1880).

* Besides the Essays to which the titles more especially refer, these volumes contain Essays on the 'Work of Volunteers in the Organisation of Charity,' 'District Visiting,' 'A Few Words to Volunteer Visitors among the Poor,' 'A More Excellent Way of Charity,' &c.

TRADE UNIONS: their Origin and Objects, Influence and Efficacy. By WILLIAM TRANT. London: Kegan Paul, Trench & Co., 1 Paternoster Square (1884).

THE ENGLISH POOR: a Sketch of their Social and Economic History; and an attempt to estimate the influence of private property on character and habit. By THOMAS MACKAY. John Murray, Albemarle Street (1889).

A HISTORY OF VAGRANTS AND VAGRANCY AND BEGGARS AND BEGGING. By C. J. RIBTON TURNER. London: Chapman & Hall (1889).

DISPAUPERISATION: a popular treatise on Poor Law evils and their remedies. By J. R. PRETYMAN, M.A. Second Edition. Longmans, Green, & Co. (1878).

PAUPERISM: ITS CAUSES AND REMEDIES. By HENRY FAWCETT, M.A., M.P., Professor of Political Economy to the University of Cambridge. London and New York: Macmillan & Co. (1871).

CHARITY ORGANISATION. By C. S. LOCH. London: Swan, Sonnenschein & Co., Paternoster Square (1890).

II.—POOR LAW AND OTHER BOOKS OF REFERENCE.

A HISTORY OF THE ENGLISH POOR LAW. By Sir GEORGE NICHOLLS, K.C.B., late Poor Law Commissioner and Secretary to the Poor Law Board. London: John Murray, Albemarle Street (1854).

THE ENGLISH POOR LAW SYSTEM PAST AND PRESENT. By Dr. P. F. ASCHROTT, Prussian District Judge; translated by HERBERT THOMAS, with a Preface by HENRY SIDGWICK, Knightbridge Professor of Moral Philosophy in the University of Cambridge. London: Knight & Co., 90 Fleet Street, E.C. (1888).

THE POOR LAW. By T. W. FOWLE, M.A., Rector of Islip. London: Macmillan & Co. (1881).

This is one of the 'English Citizen' Series, other volumes of which, dealing with the National Budget, Trade, Local Government, &c., may be found useful.

POOR LAW CONFERENCES: Current opinions, criticism, and suggestions in regard to many questions of Poor Law administration will be found in the Reports of Poor Law Conferences. London: Knight & Co.

THE POOR LAW GUARDIAN: his powers and duties in the right execution of his office. Third Edition. By WILLIAM W. MACKENZIE, M.A. Shaw & Sons, Fetter Lane (1893).

THE STATUTES IN FORCE RELATING TO THE POOR LAWS. From 43 Eliz., c. 2, to 53 Vict., c. 5 (1889); with Digests of Decisions. Two vols. by WM. CUNNINGHAM GLEN; and two vols. by Messrs. ALEX. MACMORRAN and M. S. J. MACMORRAN. London: Shaw & Sons, Fetter Lane (1873).

POOR LAW GENERAL ORDERS: being 'Orders issued by the Local Government Board and their predecessors under the Acts relating to the relief of the poor, the Elementary Education Act 1876, and the Vaccination Acts 1867, 1871, and 1874,' by ALEX. MACMORRAN and S. G. LUSHINGTON. Shaw & Sons, Fetter Lane (1890).

THE POOR LAW; comprising the whole of the Law of Relief and Settlement, and Removal of the Poor, &c. By J. F. ARCHBOLD, Esq. Twelfth Edition, by W. CUNNINGHAM GLEN, Esq. London: Shaw & Sons, Fetter Lane (1885).

THE BETTER ADMINISTRATION OF THE POOR LAW. (Charity Organisation Series.) By W. CHANCE. London: Swan, Sonnenschein & Co., 5s. net (1895).

REPORT ON POOR LAW ADMINISTRATION IN LONDON; with special
reference to the Disposal by Boards of Guardians of Applications for Relief.
By HENRY LONGLEY, Local Government Inspector (1873).

KNIGHT'S GUIDE TO THE ARRANGEMENT AND CONSTRUCTION OF
WORKHOUSE BUILDINGS. With Notes and Diagrams of the Requirements and Recommendations of the Local Government Board in regard to
the Erection of Poor Law Institutions. London: Knight & Co. (1889).

REPORT ON OUTDOOR RELIEF. By EDMOND H. WODEHOUSE, Esq., Poor
Law Inspector (1872).

CHILDREN OF THE STATE. By FLORENCE DAVENPORT HILL. Edited by
FANNY FOWKE. London : Macmillan & Co. (1889).

POOR LAWS IN FOREIGN COUNTRIES: Reports communicated to the
Local Government Board by H.M. Secretary of State for Foreign Affairs,
with Introductory Remarks by ANDREW DOYLE, Esq., Local Government Inspector (1875).

   A short Summary of these Reports, and of Information furnished in the
similar Collection edited by Emminghaus, has been published by Miss L. Twining
under the title ' Poor Relief in Foreign Countries and Outdoor Relief in England.'
London : Cassell & Co. (1889). Price 1s.

REPORTS ON THE ELBERFELD POOR-LAW SYSTEM AND GERMAN
WORKMEN'S COLONIES. By J. S. DAVY, Local Government Board;
C. S. LOCH, Secretary of the London Charity Organisation Society; and
A. F. HANEWINKEL, of the Liverpool Central Relief and Charity Organisation
Society. Eyre & Spottiswoode, East Harding Street, Fleet Street, E.C.
Price 9d.

THE COUNTY COUNCILLOR'S GUIDE: being a Handbook to the Local
Government Act 1888 and the various Provisions of the Municipal
Corporations and other Acts incorporated with it. Edited by HENRY
HOBHOUSE, M.P., and E. L. FANSHAWE. London: W. Maxwell & Son,
8 Bell Yard, Temple Bar (1888).

LONDON GOVERNMENT UNDER THE LOCAL GOVERNMENT ACT
1888. By J. F. B. FIRTH, LL.B., M.P., and EDGAR R. SIMPSON, LL.M., M.A.
London : Knight & Co., 90 Fleet Street, E.C. (1888).

THE LOCAL GOVERNMENT ACT 1894: forming an Epitome of the Law
relating to Parish Councils, and showing the alteration in the Law relating to
District Councils and Boards of Guardians. Second Edition. By ALEXANDER
MACMORRAN, M.A., and T. R. COLQUHOUN DILL, B.A. London: Shaw & Sons,
Fetter Lane (1894).

LOCAL GOVERNMENT AND LOCAL TAXATION IN ENGLAND AND
WALES. Second Edition. By HENRY HOBHOUSE, M.P., and E. L. FAN-
SHAWE. London : Sweet & Maxwell, Limited, 3 Chancery Lane (1894).

A TREATISE ON HYGIENE AND PUBLIC HEALTH. Edited by THOMAS
STEVENSON, M.D., and SHIRLEY F. MURPHY. In 3 vols. Vol. III. 'Sanitary
Law.' London: J. & A. CHURCHILL. (1894).

THE EDUCATION ACTS MANUAL. Fifteenth Edition. By HUGH OWEN.
London: Knight & Co., Fleet Street (1881).

THE FACTORY AND WORKSHOP ACT 1878. With Introduction by
ALEXANDER REDGRAVE, Esq., C.B., Her Majesty's Inspector of Factories, &c.
Third Edition. London: Shaw & Sons, Fetter Lane (1855).

THE LAW OF CHARITIES AND MORTMAIN. Being a Third Edition of Tudor's 'Charitable Trusts.' By L. S. Bristowe and Walter I. Cook. London: Reeves & Turner (1889).

THE JUSTICE'S NOTE-BOOK. By the late W. Knox Wigram. Fifth Edition, by Walter S. Shirley, M.P. London: Stevens & Sons, 119 Chancery Lane (1888).

THE JUSTICE'S MANUAL; or Guide to the Ordinary Duties of a Justice of the Peace. By the late Samuel Stone, Esq. Twenty-seventh Edition, edited by George B. Kennett, Esq. London: Shaw & Sons (1893).

— —

THE PROVIDENT KNOWLEDGE PAPERS. By George C. T. Bartley. On Pensions, Insuring One's Life, Penny Banks, Pawnbrokers, &c.

THE POST OFFICE GUIDE. Published quarterly, giving information about Savings Banks, Insurances and Annuities. Price 6d.

SOME PUBLICATIONS OF THE CHARITY ORGANISATION SOCIETY.

To be obtained at the Office of the Society and through all Booksellers

1. —Some General Papers.

ANNUAL REPORTS OF THE COUNCIL FROM 1875 TO 1893. Price 6d each.

MANUAL, CONTAINING A LIST OF THE DISTRICT COMMITTEES AND THEIR MODE OF OPERATION. Gratis.

THE CHARITY ORGANISATION PAPERS: PAPERS ON THE CONSTITUTION AND METHODS OF WORK OF THE SOCIETY:—

1. Objects, Constitution, and Method of the Charity Organisation Society.
2. Charity Organisation and Relief: a paper of Suggestions for Charity Organisation Societies.
3. The Relief of Distress.
4. Suggested Rules and Byelaws of a Charity Organisation Committee.
5. Principles of Decision.
6. Assistance by Loan.
7. Suppression of Mendicity.
8. Office Work: Books and Forms.
9. On the Accounts of District Committees.
10. Annual Reports of Charity Organisation Committees.
11. Exceptional Distress.
13. Regulations for the Conduct of Inquiry at the Offices of the Council of the London Charity Organisation Society.
14. Lists of Publications.
16. Memorandum on Out-of-work Cases.
17. Rules and Suggestions in regard to Pensions.
18. Reference of Exceptional Cases to the Administrative Committee.
19. Resolutions regarding Finance and Organisation.

II.—Papers on Charity Organisation.

CHARITY ORGANISATION. By C. S. Loch. (Social Science Series.) Price 2s. 6d.

REPORT ON THE PERSONAL VISITATION OF THE POOR (1877). Price 1d.

REPORT OF THE SUB-COMMITTEE OF THE WHITECHAPEL COMMITTEE OF THE C.O.S. ON LOCAL CHARITIES (1878).

REPORT OF THE MIGRATION SUB-COMMITTEE OF THE ST. GEORGE (HANOVER SQUARE) COMMITTEE OF THE C.O.S. (1872).

THE PREPARATION AND AUDIT OF ACCOUNTS OF CHARITABLE INSTITUTIONS. Report of a Special Committee of the Society (1890). Price 1s.

THE EFFECTS OF CHARITIES. Illustrated (1882). Price 1d.

THE DWELLINGS OF THE POOR. By C. S. Loch (1883). Price 3d.

HELPFUL WORK. By a Member of the Chelsea C.O. Committee. Price 2d.

THE CHARITY THAT IS KIND. By C. S. Loch. Price 1d.

THE FUTURE OF CHARITY. By C. S. Loch. Price 1d.

THE UNCHARITABLENESS OF INADEQUATE RELIEF. By Franc Peek (1879). Price 1d.

THE C.O.S. IN PROVINCIAL TOWNS. By J. Whitcombe, Hon. Sec Gloucester C.O.S. (1882). Price 1d.

SOME NECESSARY REFORMS IN CHARITABLE WORK. By C. S. Loch (1882).

REGISTRATION OF APPLICANTS FOR CHARITABLE ASSISTANCE. By J. T. Strang, Secretary of the Glasgow Charity Organisation Society (1883).

THE PREPARATION AND AUDIT OF THE ACCOUNTS OF CHARITABLE INSTITUTIONS. By Gérard Van de Linde, F.C.A. (1888). Price 6d.

THOROUGH CHARITY. By Miss H. Dendy (1893).

ENQUIRY AND OFFICE WORK. By H. L. Woollcombe (1893).

EMPLOYMENT OF VOLUNTEERS. By H. V. Toynbee (1893).

THE 'FRIENDLY VISITOR' AT BOSTON, U.S.A. By Miss A. H. Thwing (1893).

THE ADEQUATE TREATMENT OF TEMPORARY DISTRESS. By the Rev. L. R. Phelps (1894). Price 1d.

				Price.
CHARITY ORGANISATION . . .	Occasional Paper	1		1d.
ON SELECTING THE BEST CHARITY .	,,	,,	2	,,
ON BEGGING-LETTER WRITERS . .	,,	,,	4	,,
COMMITTEES OF MANAGEMENT .	,,	,,	6	,,
CO LECTIONS OF FUNDS BY CHARITABLE INSTITUTIONS . . .	,,	,,	6	,,
WHAT WORKERS CAN DO . . .	,,	,,	9	,,
WHY I JOINED THE CHARITY ORGANISATION SOCIETY . . .	,,	,,	11	,,
THE C.O.S. (Miss O. Hill)	,,	,,	15	,,

		Price.
IS THE ADMINISTRATION OF RELIEF THE ONLY FUNCTION OF THE SOCIETY? (T. MACKAY) . . . Occasional Paper 17		1d.
THE C.O.S. (Miss O. HILL) . . . . „ „ 20		„
ORGANISATION AND LOCAL WORK . „ „ 22		„
IT IS CHEAPER . . . . . „ „ 27		„
THE REGISTRATION OF RELIEF . . „ „ 38		„
ALMSGIVING NO CHARITY (DEFOE) . „ „ 39		„
CHARITY ORGANISATION (C. S. LOCH, in Weekly Dispatch, July 1893) . . „ „ 40		„
EFFECTUAL WORK (Miss SEWELL) . . „ „ 41		„

CHARITY ORGANISATION. By the late J. HORNSBY WRIGHT (1883). Price 3d.

LONDON AND PROVINCIAL ASPECTS OF CHARITY ORGANISATION. By M. W. MOGGRIDGE, Esq. (1881). Price 1d.

A FEW FACTS AND REFLECTIONS CONCERNING THE ST. MARYLE-BONE INQUIRY BOOK. Compiled, for that District Committee of the Society, by O. H. (1870). Price 1d.

THE PROVINCIAL REGISTER. A Register of Provincial Charity Organisation and Relief Societies in correspondence with the London C.O.S., containing Summaries of the last Annual Reports of nearly 100 British Societies, with their Officers, Hours, and Methods of Work; also a List of Colonial and Foreign Societies, and other information. Price 6d.

III.—THE CHARITY ORGANISATION SOCIETY AND THE CLERGY.

A SCHEME FOR A PAROCHIAL RELIEF COMMITTEE. By the late G. CHARLES. Price 6d.

THE ORGANISATION OF RELIEF IN THE PARISH. By the Rev. C. E. BROOKE. (Occasional Paper 16.) Price 1d.

THE CLERGY AND RELIEF. By the Rev. H. MEYER. (Occasional Paper 18.) Price 1d.

THE SCIENCE OF CHARITY. By the ARCHBISHOP OF CANTERBURY. (Occasional Paper 19.) Price 1d.

THE CHARITIES OF CHURCH AND CHAPEL. (Occasional Paper 23.) Price 1d.

DISTRICT VISITING. By Miss O. HILL. (Occasional Paper 28.) Price 1d.

CHURCH CHARITY: a Good Example. (Occasional Paper 37.) Price 1d.

CHARITY ORGANISATION AND CHURCH AGENCIES: Papers read by the Hon and Rev. W. H. FREEMANTLE and the Rev. S. A. BARNETT (1880). Price 1d.

IV.—THE CHARITY ORGANISATION SOCIETY AND THE POOR LAW.

THREE LETTERS TO THE TIMES, with Leading Article, &c., on 'London Pauperism.' By the late Sir CHARLES TREVELYAN (1870). Price 6d.

VOLUNTARY VERSUS LEGAL RELIEF. By the Rev. R. J. PRETTYMAN (1879) Price 1d.

CO-OPERATION OF CHARITABLE AGENCIES WITH THE POOR LAW. By T. Mackay (1893). Price 1d.

FROM PAUPERISM TO MANLINESS. By the late T. Bland Garland. (Occasional Paper 21.) Price 1d.

RELIEF OF THE POOR IN THE METROPOLIS : a Minute of the Poor Law Board (1869). (Occasional Paper 24.) Price 1d.

OUTDOOR RELIEF. By T. Mackay. (Occasional Paper 33.) Price 1d.

WHY IS IT WRONG TO SUPPLEMENT OUTDOOR RELIEF? (Occasional Paper 31.) Price 1d.

THE INTEREST OF THE WORKING-CLASS IN THE POOR LAW. By T. Mackay. (Occasional Paper 34.) Price 1d.

THE TRUE POLICY OF POOR RELIEF. (Occasional Paper 43.) Price 1d.

RELIEF IN KIND TO THE OUTDOOR POOR. By a Metropolitan Relieving Officer. Price 1d.

STATE ORGANISATION AND VOLUNTARY AID. By Miss L. Twining. (1882). Price 1d.

V.—Papers on Medical Relief.

MEMORANDUM ON THE MEDICAL CHARITIES OF THE METRO-POLIS, with special reference to the proposal for an inquiry in regard to the administration and common organisation of Voluntary Hospitals and Dispensaries, and Poor Law Infirmaries and Dispensaries by a Select Committee of the House of Lords (1889). Price 1s.

INTERIM REPORT OF A SPECIAL COMMITTEE FOR PROMOTING AN INQUIRY BY THE HOUSE OF LORDS ON THE MANAGEMENT AND COMMON ORGANISATION OF MEDICAL CHARITIES OF THE METROPOLIS; with Notes of Evidence. By Lieut.-Col. Montefiore, R.A. (1890). Price 1s.

FINAL REPORT OF ABOVE COMMITTEE (1892). Price 6d.

METROPOLITAN MEDICAL RELIEF. Read by the late Sir Charles Trevelyan at a Conference presided over by Dr. Acland, with Remarks by the late Sir Wm. Gull, Bart., Mr. Prescott Hewett, Sir Rutherford Alcock, and others. With Appendices. (Revised 1880.) Price 6d.

Contents of Appendices :

1. Report on the Social Position of the Out-Patients of the Royal Free Hospital.
2. The Limits of Unpaid Service.
3. First Report of the Medical Committee of the Charity Organisation Society.
4. Revised Model Rules for Provident Dispensaries (June 1878), by the Medical Committee of the Charity Organisation Society.
5. Correspondence relating to the Memorial to the British Medical Association.
6. Speeches delivered by the late Sir William Gull, Bart.

REPORTS OF THE COMMITTEES AND SUB-COMMITTEES of Members of the Medical Profession in London, appointed to inquire into the subject of Out-Patient Hospital Administration in the Metropolis (1871). Price 1s.

THE EXTENSION OF PROVIDENT DISPENSARIES THROUGHOUT LONDON AND ITS ENVIRONS. Read by the late Sir Charles Trevelyan before a Special Meeting of the Charity Organisation Society, presided over by the late Lord Frederick Cavendish, M.P. (1878). Price 1d.

THE DOCTOR'S BILL, OR NO DOCTOR'S BILL. A Word to Working Men and their Families (1878). Price 1d.

OUT-PATIENT REFORM, including Letters to the *Times* from Mr. Timothy Holmes, Mr. T. Fowell Buxton, the late Sir Charles Trevelyan, and the Rev. Canon Erskine Clarke; and a Speech by the late Sir William Gull (1878). Price 3d.

CROSS-PURPOSES IN MEDICAL REFORM: a Paper read by C. S. Loch, Secretary to the Charity Organisation Society (1885). Price 2d.

VI.—Reports and Papers on the Distribution of Food and Free Feeding.

CHARITY AND FOOD. The Report of a Special Committee of the Society upon Soup Kitchens, Children's Breakfasts and Dinners, and Cheap Food Supply; with Evidence (1887). Price 1s.

REPORT ON SOUP KITCHENS (1877). Price 3d.

A SOUP KITCHEN IN ST. GILES'S: a Report by the St. Giles's Committee of the Society on the Condition and Character of Recipients of Soup Relief in January 1879. Price 3d.

FIRST REPORT OF A SPECIAL COMMITTEE OF THE SOCIETY appointed to consider the best means of dealing with School Children alleged to be in Want of Food (January 1891). Price 6d.

THE BETTER WAY OF ASSISTING SCHOOL CHILDREN: a Report on Experiments in the Organisation of Charity for the better Assistance of School Children, with Suggestions and Recommendations (1893). Price 2s. 6d.

THE SCHOOL BOARD AND CHILDREN IN WANT OF FOOD: a Reprint of a Letter to the *Times* (December 1889).

THE FEEDING OF ADULTS. (Occasional Paper 13.) Price 1d.

THE FEEDING OF SCHOOL CHILDREN. (Occasional Paper 14.) Price 1d.

THE ASSISTANCE OF SCHOOL CHILDREN. By Mrs. Leon. (Occasional Paper 45.)

VII.—Reports and Papers regarding Homeless Cases and Street Mendicancy.

CONFERENCE ON NIGHT REFUGES AND REPORT OF COMMITTEE (1870). Price 4d.

REPORT ON THE EMPLOYMENT OF ITALIAN CHILDREN FOR MENDICANT AND IMMORAL PURPOSES. By a Special Committee of the Society. Second Edition, enlarged. With appendix, and report of a deputation to the Home Secretary (1877). Price 1s.

REPORT OF THE SPECIAL COMMITTEE ON HOMELESS CASES. With evidence (1891). Price 1s.

INVESTIGATION IN SOME OF ITS FEATURES. By the late J. Hornsby Wright (1872). Price 2d.

BEGGARS AND IMPOSTORS. By the late J. Hornsby Wright (1883). Price 2d.

THE PLAGUE OF BEGGARS. By the late Dr. Guy (1868). Price 1d.

THE NUISANCE OF STREET MUSIC. By the late Dr. Guy (1868). Price 1d.

STARVATION CASES. Reprinted from letters published in the *Times* (December 1892). Price 1d.

VIII.—REPORTS AND PAPERS ON WANT OF EMPLOYMENT AND EXCEPTIONAL DISTRESS.

REPORT ON THE BEST MEANS OF DEALING WITH EXCEPTIONAL DISTRESS. By a Special Committee of the Society; with evidence (November 1886). Price 6d.

THE DUTCH HOME LABOUR COLONIES: their Origin and Development. By H. G. WILLINK (1889). Price 1s. 6d.

UNSKILLED LABOUR AND RELIEF WORKS. By Sir S. G. JOHNSON (1894). Price 1d.

MUNICIPAL WORKSHOPS. By the late Dr. BRADBY. (Occasional Paper 29.) Price 1d.

THE UNEMPLOYED. By H. C. BOURNE. (Occasional Paper 30.) Price 1d.

FIRST REPORT OF THE MANSION HOUSE CONFERENCE ON THE CONDITION OF THE UNEMPLOYED (November 1887 to July 1888). Price 6d.

THE STATE AND THE UNEMPLOYED; with Notes regarding the Action of Vestries in different parts of London (1892-93). Price 3d.

IX.—REPORTS AND PAPERS ON THE AFFLICTED.

INTERIM REPORT OF SPECIAL COMMITTEE ON THE FEEBLE-MINDED, EPILEPTIC, DEFORMED, AND CRIPPLED. With statistical tables (1891). Price 2s. 6d.

THE FEEBLE-MINDED CHILD AND ADULT: a Report on an Investigation of the Physical and Mental Condition of 50,000 School Children, with Suggestions for the better Education and Care of Feeble-minded Children and Adults (1893). Price 2s. 6d.

THE EPILEPTIC AND CRIPPLED CHILD AND ADULT: a Report on the Present Condition of these Classes of Afflicted Persons, with Suggestions for their better Education and Employment (1893). Price 2s. 6d.

X.—ON THE BLIND.

REPORT ON THE TRAINING OF THE BLIND. By a Special Committee of the Society; with Appendix (1878). Price 1s.

THE TRAINING OF THE BLIND: Extracts from the first European Congress of Teachers of the Blind. (Vienna, August 1873.) Translated by Major-General BAISBRIGGE, R.E. (1875).

SUGGESTIONS TO THE PARENTS AND FRIENDS OF BLIND CHILDREN.

XI.—REPORTS AND PAPERS ON THRIFT.

REPORT OF SPECIAL COMMITTEE ON INSURANCE AND SAVING (Charity Organisation Series, published by Messrs. Swan Sonnenschein & Co., Paternoster Square, E.C.) (1892). Price 2s. 6d.

FRIENDLY SOCIETIES AND THE LIMITS OF STATE AID AND CONTROL IN INDUSTRIAL INSURANCE. By Sir GEORGE YOUNG, Bart., formerly Assistant Commissioner to the Friendly Societies Commission, 1870-3 (1879). Price 1d.

THE WORK OF CHARITY IN PROMOTING PROVIDENT HABITS. By G. C. T. BARTLEY, Manager of the National Penny Bank, Limited (1879). Price 1d.

THRIFT AND PROVIDENCE. By Mr. R. A. Leach (1891). Price 1d.

THREE FRIENDLY SOCIETIES. (Occasional Paper 25.) Price 1d.

A SAFE ANNUITY. (Occasional Paper 26.) Price 1d.

THE PROVIDENT FUND COLLECTOR. (Occasional Paper 32.) Price 1d.

THE COLLECTING SAVINGS BANK. (Occasional Paper 36.) Price 1d.

XII.—Pamphlets and Papers regarding Old Age and Pensions.

NATIONAL PENSIONS. By H. C. Bourne. (Occasional Paper 35.) Price 1d.

OLD-AGE PENSIONS: an Ounce of Fact. (Occasional Paper 42.) Price 1d.

PRIVATE CHARITY AND PENSIONS. (Occasional Paper 44.) Price 1d.

OLD-AGE PENSIONS AND PAUPERISM: an Enquiry as to the bearing of the Statistics of Pauperism quoted by the Right Hon. J. Chamberlain, M.P., and others in support of a Scheme for National Pensions (1892). Price 1s.

PAUPERISM AND OLD-AGE PENSIONS: a Paper read at the South Wales Poor Law Conference, 1892. By C. S. Loch. Price 6d.

THE CHARITY ORGANISATION REVIEW.

The Official Organ of the Charity Organisation Society.

Principally addressed to persons interested in charitable work.

It contains articles on social and economic subjects, charity and the Poor Law, and notes on current matters relating to artisans' dwellings, industrial insurance, thrift, Poor Law administration, charitable institutions, &c. The proceedings of the Council are published in it, with notes respecting the work of charity organisation in the provinces and abroad. It contains also reviews of books, short abstracts of Blue Books, Parliamentary Papers, &c., which may be useful to almoners for purposes of reference.

Published 1st of each month, price 6d., or sent, post free, for 6s. 6d. per annum.

Back numbers of the REVIEW, from 1885 to date, can be obtained on application.

TABLE OF CONTENTS
OF
CHARITIES REGISTER AND DIGEST.*
FOURTH EDITION (1895).

* Published by the Charity Organisation Society, 15 Buckingham Street, London, W.C., and Longmans, Green, & Co.

APPENDIX.